THIS ISN'T
BRAVE

Publisher
Balthazar Pagani

Editorial assistant
PEPE *nymi*

Graphic design
Davide Canesi / PEPE *nymi*

© 2022 White Star s.r.l.
Piazzale Luigi Cadorna, 6 – 20123 Milan, Italy
www.whitestar.it

Translation: ICEIGeo, Milan (translation: Alexa Ahern)
Editing: Phillip Gaskill

Copyright © 2022 by Laetitia Duveau.
Published by Mango Publishing, a division of Mango Publishing
Group, Inc.
Library of Congress Cataloging-in-Publication number: 2022937333
ISBN: (print) 978-1-68481-039-0 \ (ebook) 978-1-68481-040-6

THIS ISN'T

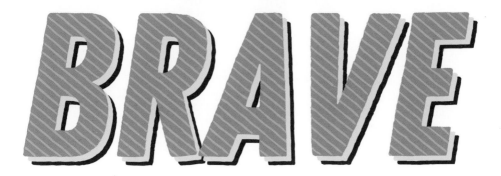

BRAVE

A BRAVE GIRL'S GUIDE TO
BODY POSITIVITY & SELF-ACCEPTANCE

Laetitia Duveau

Illustrations by
Bridget Moore

Edited by
Caterina Grimaldi

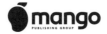
mango
PUBLISHING GROUP

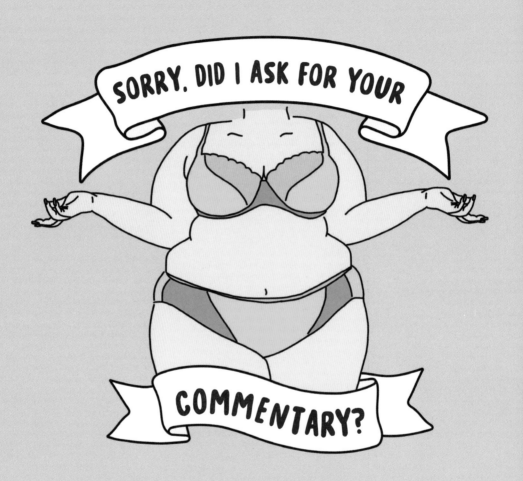

CONTENTS

• • • • •

A NEW KIND OF FEMININITY

My name is Laetitia Duveau, and I am the founder of **Curated By GIRLS**, a platform I started in Berlin in 2016 to promote **diversity** through art with a focus on **femininity**. Being an artist myself (a musician), I wanted to offer a free space to highlight the work of women and non-binary artists, to help those who feel alone, misunderstood, judged, or exposed.

Inclusivity is important in helping us build our sense of self, and the tools needed to sustain inclusivity must be accessible because not everyone lives in big cities. Some of us live in isolated places or in very closed-off or discriminatory environments where it is almost impossible to live authentically as ourselves. I know what it means to be excluded, to not have the space to be listened to. When I was offered the opportunity to write a guide to self-acceptance, I accepted the challenge.

I am not an expert in sociology or psychology, but every day since 2016, I have looked through visual materials from emerging artists in every part of the world—and the comments that come with them, even hostile ones—and they have given me a clear view of what society is like today.

We are at a turning point in our evolution. It seems that we should seriously think about a system based less on social success and more on self-actualization, which can sometimes feel like it's a million miles from what we should be. Recently, I have understood that the ego we are constantly urged to awaken—the one that buys things compulsively, that is jealous, keeps us stuck in our own heads—quite often falls prey to a masculine mentality and doesn't necessarily correspond to our inner self.

With this book, which has been brilliantly illustrated by the talented Bridget Moore (a.k.a. **Handsome Girl**), I would like to help young women and girls feel better about themselves and feel strong. Everyone feels pain, to different degrees, and if I can't change the world, I can at least try to do some good and offer simple ideas for feeling better about ourselves.

Addressing all these very important concepts in such a limited space was a challenge. On the other hand, conciseness made it lighter and more accessible—and we all need a bit of levity, don't you think? One of my mottos is "Do things seriously without taking yourself too seriously."

Oh, yes, I almost forgot. Even if I'm mostly speaking to women, anyone can read this book. It is very enriching to attempt to understand someone who's different from us, so reading it to the people around us (even the most resistant) could maybe help them better understand the world we live in.

I hope you enjoy reading along with me, without prejudice and hopefully with a smile. And if this guide is useful, then . . . mission accomplished.

Did you know that in Latin, *laetitia* means "joy?" :)

Be strong, Babes!

Laetitia Duveau

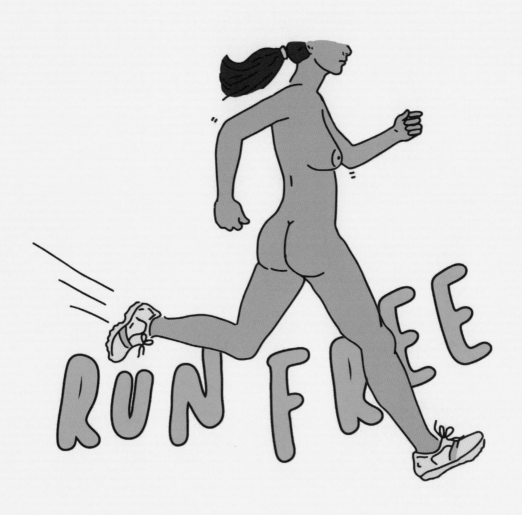

Chapter 1

· · · · ·

Your Body Is Yours Alone

· · · · ·

The body. You know, that thing that follows us everywhere but that we know so little about. Exploring our anatomy is the starting point to knowing who we are. The site of many battles and the origin of many taboos, the body is more than anything a place where the defense of our rights starts. It is our home, and our decisions regarding it are ours alone.

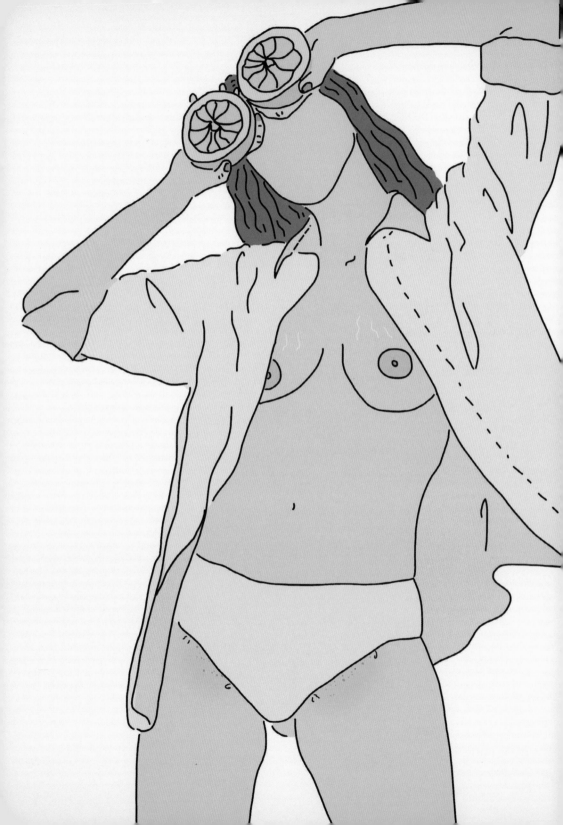

HANDS OFF MY NIPPLES

Oh, nipples! Those little spots of skin that are always making news. If you had told me that one day my nipples would have been censored, I wouldn't have believed you! Most mammals have nipples, and yet our cultural system, which claims to be "evolved," has two standards. It has decided that female nipples are FIRST AND FOREMOST a sexual object, and therefore must be covered up, even for breastfeeding.

Male nipples can be shown without issue. Ours, on the other hand, are offensive! This communicates a sexual message! Even on social media, female nipples are absolutely FORBIDDEN from being published, unless you want to risk losing your account, which has triggered a full-on nipple hunt.

It's very offensive that the female body is constantly censored and reported. Social media should truly represent us and help us feel good about ourselves, not perpetuate the endless sexualization of our bodies.

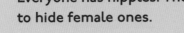

#STOPCENSORINGWOMENSBODIES

#BORNTHISWAY   #FREENIPPLE

#MYNIPPLESEXIST

Everyone has nipples. There's no reason to hide female ones.

CLIT, CLIT, HOORAY!

Did you know that the clitoris is the nerve center of female pleasure? The organ is much more important than it seems—or, rather, than they wanted us to believe. For a long time, the clitoris was considered an evil thing, and it was often even removed (which still happens in some cultures). Why? It would seem that female pleasure was seen as a threat to society. Just reading that sentence gives me goose bumps.

But finally we know. The clitoris can have an infinite number of shapes and colors, and it is the only organ in the human body intended exclusively for pleasure.

We can look at it, even admire it. Will it bite? No? Oh, good! And no doubt remains: all orgasms come from sensations that spread from this area. So, ladies, ready, set . . . go!

#NICETOMEETYOU   #CLITCLITCLIT

#KNOWYOURSELF   #NOTABOOS

Get a mirror, take a look at your clitoris, and don't be afraid. Enjoy!

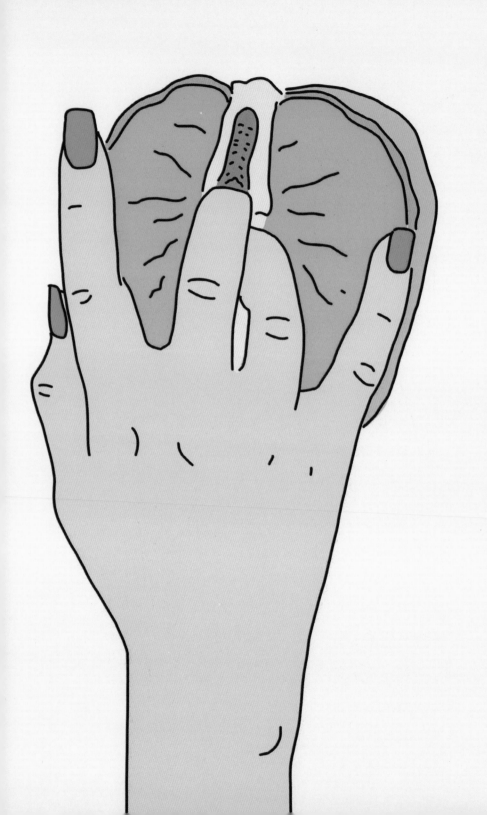

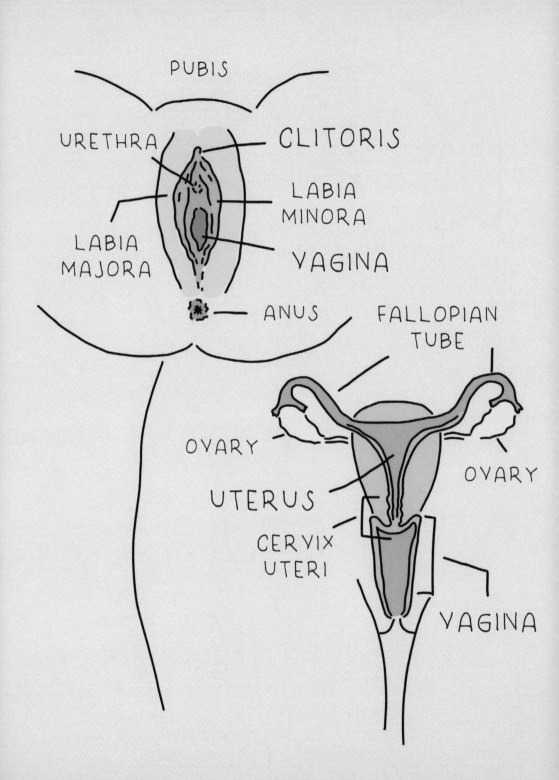

THE VAGINA: ONE PART OF A WHOLE

If we are speaking of anatomy in a strict sense, the vagina is the channel that connects the external genitals to the uterus. It is part of the female reproductive system, and it enables penetration during sexual intercourse. Not only that, but it also allows sperm to reach the uterus for fertilization and lets menstrual flow exit. And this magic system is self-cleaning, thanks to its white discharge. Incredible!

But the vagina is also an organ of desire of all types, especially for people with male genitals. Since heterosexual men reach orgasm essentially by rubbing against the vagina, today we realize that women were defined sexually according to that which provokes pleasure in MEN. That's why for so long the entire female sexual organ was called by the name of only one of its parts. OMG, how could we have let this happen? "Vagina" and "vulva" are two different things. Once again, thanks to the patriarchy for this confusion!

#VMAGIC   #THEVAGINAISNTHEVULVA
#WELCOMETOMYVAGINA

Calling each part of our body by its name shouldn't be such a challenge.

17

VIVA LA VULVA

Vul-va! What a funny, simple little word. Yet, in our binary/patriarchal culture, it is almost difficult to say. Or shameful! And thus, our poor vulvas have been and continue to be victims of many taboos and censorship, to the point that it is often confused with the vagina, the internal channel. The vulva is the external part of our genitals, and it includes the pubis, labia, clitoris, openings of the urethra and vagina, and the area up to the anus. So many spots to explore! So, where does the confusion come from, you might ask? The error derives from the fact that female anatomy was for a long time studied in terms of its role "for" cisgender, heterosexual men, rather than as independent organs. Thus, by ignoring the names of various parts of our genitals and seeing women depicted with nothing between their legs, we have forgotten to familiarize ourselves with our bodies, forgotten our pleasure to the point that we find our vulvas ugly, strange, and abnormal. . . . Obviously, if we continue to not look at it or name it, it becomes a mysterious monster! Some have even chosen the scalpel to reduce its size, shape, and labia, a serious trend that sends shivers down my back. Well...really down my vulva! Rest assured; your vulva is normal. It's beautiful. All vulvas are beautiful in their diversity. I insist. Artists are creating more and more art in its image, restoring its former glory. Hallelujah!

#CELEBRATEVULVA **#VULVALANDSCAPE**
#MYVULVAISBEAUTIFUL

Let us celebrate all vulvas, marvelous landscapes waiting to be explored.

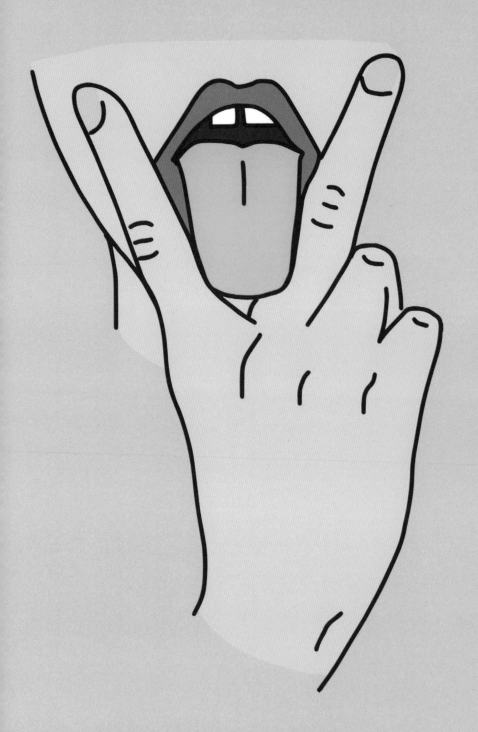

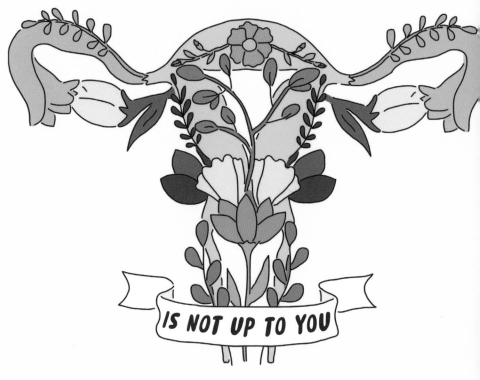

UTERINDEPENDENCE

The uterus. "The womb of life" from which we all come. This organ is all about reproduction, but today, reproducing isn't very "glam." We are emancipated and live outside the walls of domestic life. We aren't baby mills. However, the uterus still finds itself as the physical center of the patriarchal system, as if it were the most important characteristic of femininity. And cis men who don't have one are very interested in the uterus. Or rather they are very interested in controlling everything that happens inside of it. That's why in some countries we still have to fight for the fundamental right to decide for our body, and we must never let our guard down when it comes to defending our rights. Having a uterus should give us the freedom to choose whether we want a child or not. Because the uterus belongs exclusively to the person who has one. And no one else. Period.

As for me, I discovered I have two uteri. It's called a uterus didelphys. The more the merrier!

#IMINCHARGEOFMYUTERUS

#MYUTERUSMYCHOICE

#NOUTERUSNOOPINION

No uterus, no opinion.

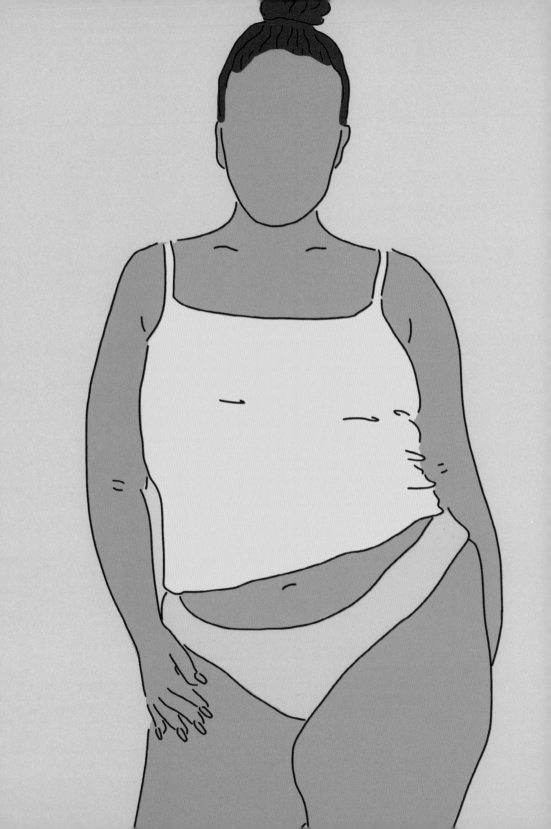

Chapter 2

. . . . .

Real
Bodies

. . . . .

We don't always love our curves. Often, we want to change
our bodies, and it can take a lifetime to accept ourselves
as we are. This is especially true within the world of social
media, where we unfortunately can hide behind filters, like
virtual Botox injections. The disturbing thing is that the latest
trend is to actually get surgery to resemble this so-called
perfect *fake* appearance. It's sad to live in a world in which
we are encouraged to be someone else. . . .

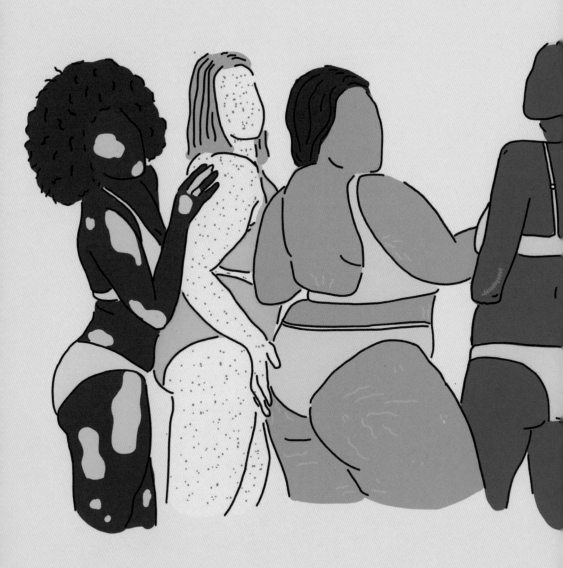

DIVERSITY = BEAUTY

The conformist and unrealistic standards we see every day put an outrageous amount of pressure on us. We are never enough, but we are also always too much—too tall, too fat, too skinny, too short, too made-up, too sexy, too much of this, too much of that—and we are constantly judged based on appearance. Enough is enough!

Let's take a deep breath and start to decide for ourselves. We are all beautiful, especially when we are comfortable with ourselves. Right? Have you ever noticed that when you feel good in your own skin, you feel more confident and alive? Beauty has everything to do with feeling good. But, of course, it's not easy in daily life. It's a personal journey.

And beauty is all around us. When we look at the world instead of spending our time judging others and ourselves, we find beauty everywhere, beauty that is stronger and more powerful than our fears, that allows us to see that everything is relative. What a relief!

#NOSTANDARDS #TOEACHTHEIROWN
#BEAUTYINALLSHAPESANDSIZES

Aesthetic standards are unrealistic, and they have no place here!

YOU ARE NOT A NUMBER ON A SCALE

You can't measure someone's worth in pounds or kilos! And yet many of us live for the number on the scale. It goes without saying that we are tortured by the matter of ideal weight and are bombarded by diet advertising! Obviously, it gets in our heads. I just want to say that we all have the right to decide what makes us feel good. But it isn't always easy to feel confident enough to listen to ourselves. And then there's this issue of medical "standards" that tell us what is "normal." Could it be part of a system that wants to sell us things? No one can force us to be a certain way, especially because we all have the ability to listen to ourselves and our bodies, leaving social pressure in the dirt.

And one other thing: Do you know what images are most often censored or removed from social media? That's right, the worst of the worst we SHOULD NOT show are fat rolls, especially female ones.

They know that seeing more representation of real women's bodies will lead to more women accepting themselves as they are. Which isn't what advertising companies are going for.

#NOIDEALWEIGHT

#MYWEIGHTISNOTMYVALUE

Your weight and clothing size are not equal to your worth.

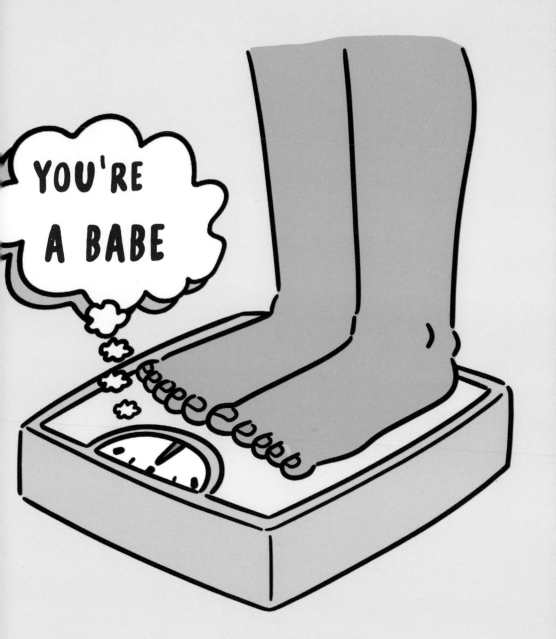

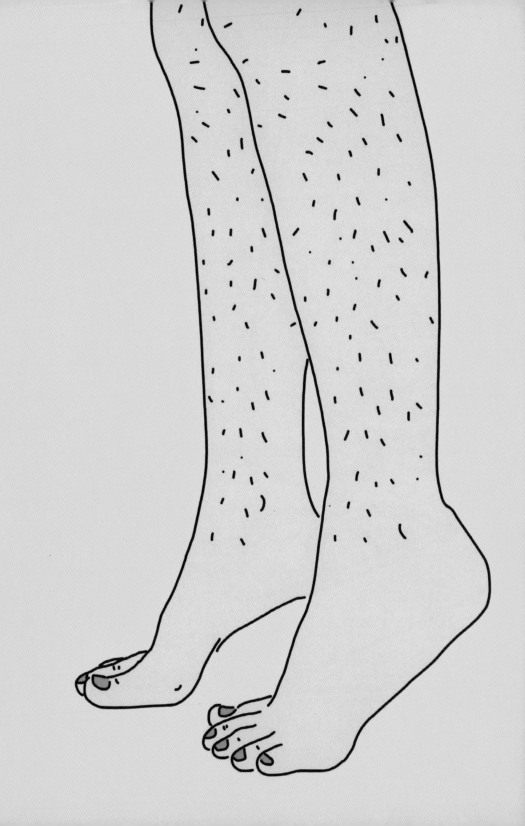

I HAVE, YOU HAVE, WE ALL HAVE HAIR

Who says hair has to be removed? Long, short, curly, straight, dyed, highlighted, or natural, hair protects us from the cold, the heat, and the dirt. You might like it or not. You might like shaving or going all natural. Like always, it's a matter of preference and should be a personal choice.

But society has made us believe that body hair is not compatible with femininity, so that they can sell us razors and hair-removal creams. So now it's not easy to show up as we like, especially in a space that makes us feel constantly judged. But let's not forget that everyone has hair, no matter their gender, and it doesn't need to be condemned or eliminated.

#HAIR   #HAIRDRESSER
#MYHAIRMYCHOICE
#LONGHAIRDONTCARE

In case you missed it: All humans have hair!
If you want to let it grow, go for it!

THE MARKS ON OUR SKIN

Perfect skin is practically a fantasy, invented by Mr. Photoshop and photo filters! A true revolution of self-deception! When a mirror appears, we instantly begin to compare ourselves with airbrushed models. Is that me? With pimples? Moles? Bags under my eyes? Noooo! And what about scars? Isn't it a shame that we don't appreciate the parts of us that have a story to tell? Sure, the marks and wrinkles remind us every day that we are aging. And, of course, that's not what we want to reflect on every time we wake up. But these "imperfections" (as we love to call them) give us character, a visible story, one that can sometimes be dramatic, but that is authentically ours. Living with these traces is not always easy, but they are a part of us. Therefore, we can spend time hating them or covering them up, but only when we accept them do we free ourselves of useless suffering and perhaps become an inspiration for someone else. That's the most powerful thing ever.

#LOVETHESKINYOUREIN

#YOURSKINYOURJOURNEY

#STOPPHOTOSHOP

Parts of our story are written on our skin.

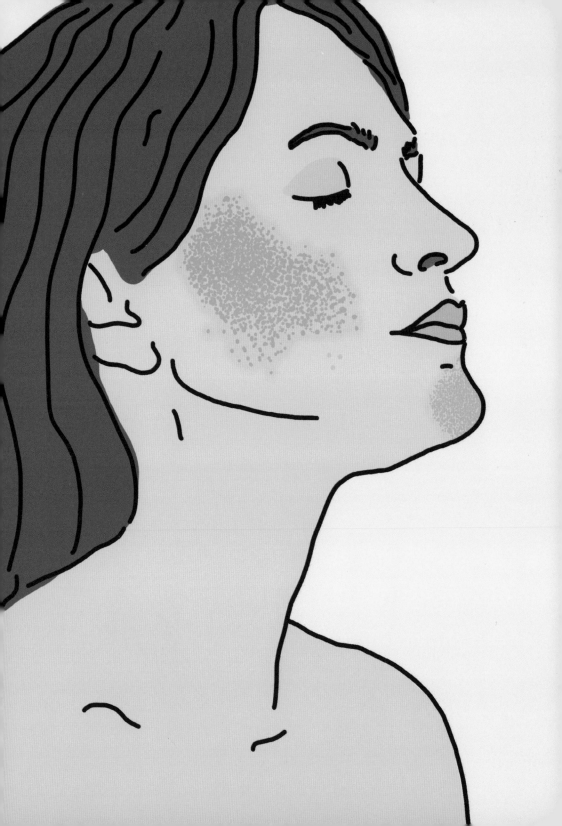

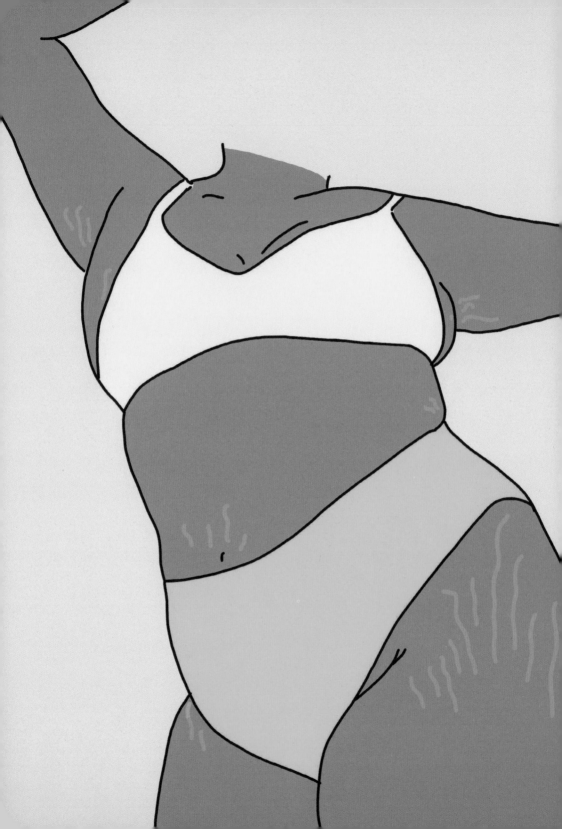

STRETCH MARKS: THE LINES OF OUR EVOLUTION

We will not repeat it: nearly everyone has stretch marks. They are like waves or the scratches of a tiger on our skin. They are a part of us, but once again, the widespread use of photo retouching makes us believe that we must eliminate them, erase them, smooth them over. But they exist, so why don't we learn to live with them? Goodbye stretch mark creams, hello freedom.

Stretch marks arise from hormonal variations or quick changes in size, like those due to growth or pregnancy, and they usually appear on areas that change the most: breasts, thighs, and hips during adolescence, breasts and stomachs during pregnancy. We can be proud of these lines that bear witness to our evolution. Yes, our bodies grow and change. Who said that our bodies must stay the same always? Change is not an illness.

#BODIESCHANGESOWHAT   #LOVEYOURLINES
#WELOVESTRETCHMARKS

"Stretch marks? Here's how to get rid of them!" they say, offering crazy ideas instilled in us from a very young age. Why not simply love them? They are part of us and our story. There's no reason to eliminate them.

CELLULITE, NO PROBLEM

Ladies, 90 percent of us have it, no matter our size. But cellulite is one of our greatest insecurities, is it not? In the seventeenth century, cellulite was a standard of beauty. Think of *The Three Graces* by Paul Rubens, the painting that clearly highlights the dimples of the three goddesses, who don't seem uncomfortable at all. So, what happened? How did we get to this point? Today, media and magazines pressure us to eliminate our cellulite.

They sell us magical creams at high prices, and, let's be honest, they don't even work. It's just a waste of money, a lost battle from the start on a purely physical level. We can kill ourselves trying to erase our cellulite, or we can use our energy for something more constructive and fun. Like defending our rights, wearing a bikini with confidence, or going to the beach and enjoying the day. Right?

#GIVEMEBACKMYMONEY   #CELLULITEISOK

#TAKEBACKTHELOTION   #OTHERBATTLES

#ALLBODIESAREGOODBODIES

**Choose your battles wisely
and fight the ones that are worth it.**

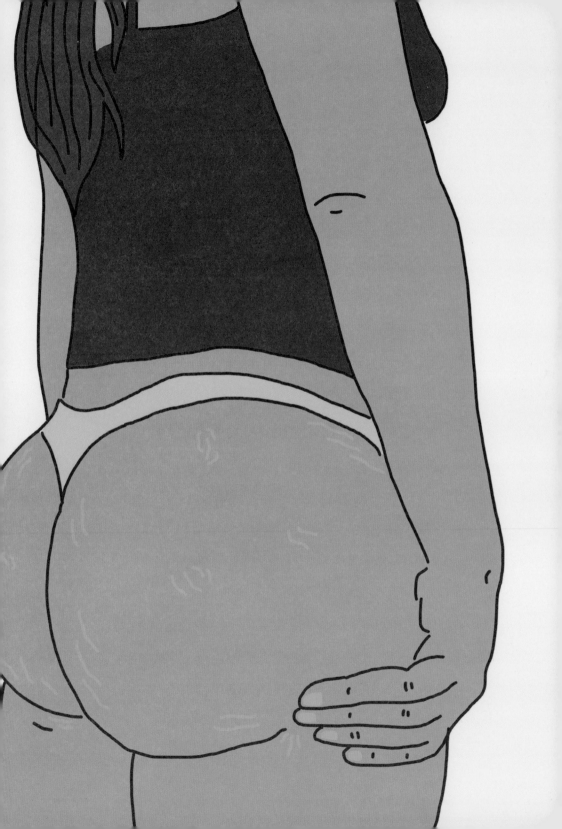

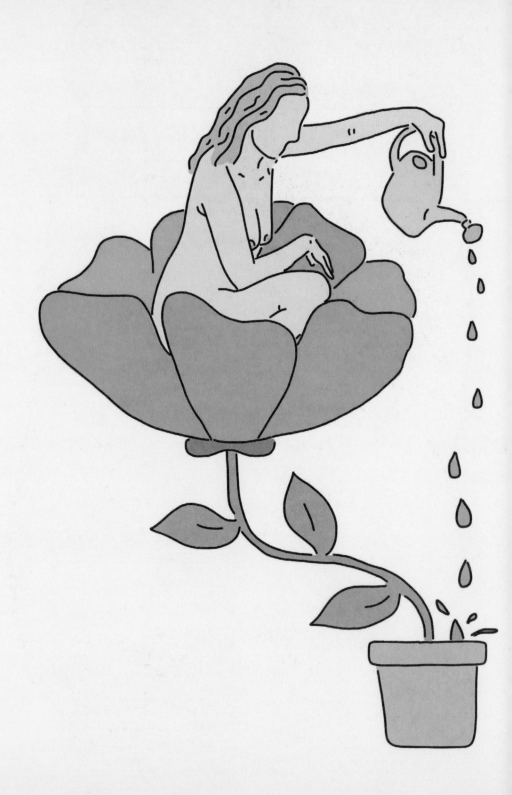

AGING AT YOUR OWN PACE

"How old are you?" It's one of the first questions we are asked when we meet someone, as if our ages could reveal our stories and define our personalities. Age puts us in a box, or should I say a cage? And what if age had little to do with the journey? Why can't you start a career at whatever age you want? Sometimes we are not psychologically ready, but we feel forced to run with the ticking of the clock. We are told what we should and shouldn't be doing at every age (although young women and girls should keep in mind their limits in terms of sexuality). For women aging means getting old, whereas for men it means maturing. How strange.

Our society is obsessed with youth, especially that of women, who are supposed to be young, unrealistically "beautiful," and . . . quiet. More than anything, society is obsessed with the youth of our bodies. C'mon, enough of this. We must respect everyone's journey.

#BANISHTHECULTOFYOUTH
#ALWAYSTOOIMPORTANT #AGE

Even if you think it's too late to do something, go for it. Now is a good time.

ME, AU NATUREL

Odor: there's coconut, mango, almond, jasmine . . . mmm . . . and then there's body odors. Like after I've almost fainted from the stress of giving a speech during a conference. Or when I've come back after a forty-five-minute walk in the midday heat. You know what I'm talking about? Let's be honest: in our society, "smelling" is a CRIME. Let's be real: we like to smell good, but wanting to be a doll that smells *only* like roses all the time is a fantasy. You can choose your perfume; you can't choose your odor. You might want to try to hide it under endless layers of deodorant. But odor is a part of us, and it changes depending on our moods. It expresses our desires, our anxieties . . . our intense emotions. It is our body speaking. I find it fascinating, don't you? So, love, or at least accept, the odor of your body without shame. This should be natural for all of us.

#PUREODOR   #THEBODYSPEAKS
#MYNATURALODOR

Let your body express itself.
Your mood determines your odor.

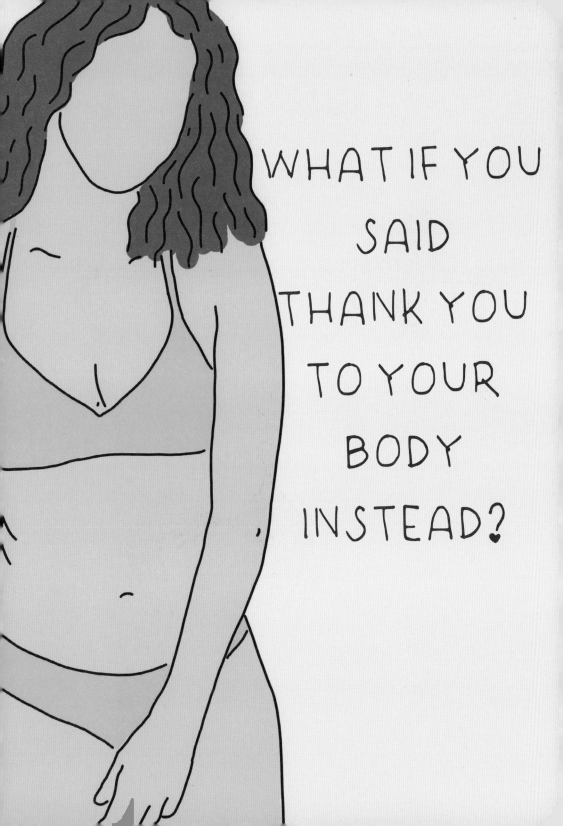

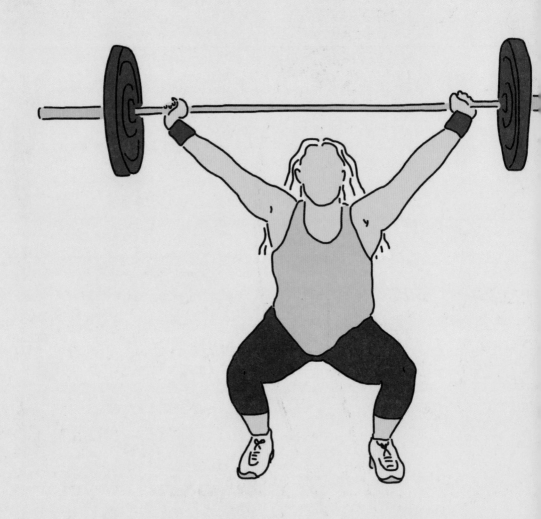

SUPER STRENGTH!

The binary on which our society is built leads us to believe in falsehoods like men are strong and women are weak. Sure, men and women have different physical characteristics, but does physical strength really belong to just one gender? Why should a woman always be represented in the same way? Young, thin, slim, silent, and (of course) not too muscular. Out of the question. Muscles are reserved for cis men!

I'm not talking about bodybuilding, but about the idea of weakness and strength. In any case, why shouldn't a woman be a bodybuilder if she wants? As for me, I believe everyone should be what they want, without others sticking their noses where they don't belong. :)

I know that physical strength is not one of my main qualities. My arms look like two long baguettes; but when I am really (really) angry, my strength doubles. Like Superwoman! Taking time to improve your strength can help you gain confidence; when you go to the gym, think about getting strong, not about losing weight.

#BRAVERTHANYOUKNOW
#STRONGERTHANYOUTHINK
#STRONGWOMEN

Women are weak and men are strong:
a stereotype that's damaging for everyone!

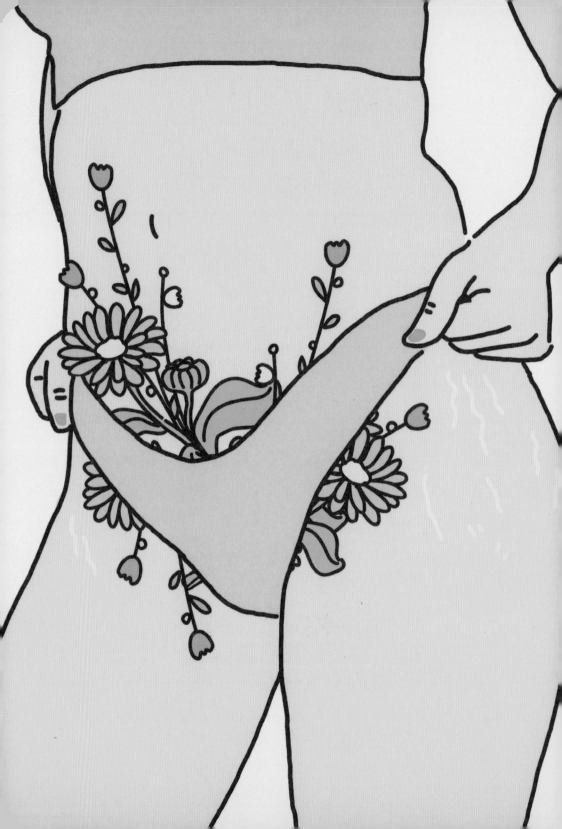

. . . . .

Chapter 3

A Spotlight on Pleasure

. . . . .

Are you in search of pleasure and your
own sexuality? Let's explore it deeper
to better understand it.

THE PERSPECTIVE OF FEMALE PLEASURE

We have been taught strange ideas about female sexuality. For example, "Can women even orgasm?" "Sex sometimes hurts for women, get used to it." or "A woman's pleasure is sinful and self-indulgent." Apparently, if we believe in the predominant narrative, female sexuality is less important than that of men. Us women are romantic but cold creatures who are just waiting for our handsome princes, whose notable presence would fill our lives enough that we don't need pleasure. We would have love, true love!

It should be noted that medicine took its time to acknowledge the presence and importance of the clitoris. This little organ (which is much larger than believed) was ignored for a long time, and only recently did we learn its true shape. Let's be honest (I say sarcastically), the vagina was specifically meant to satisfy cis, hetero men (sex machines whose pleasure is obviously more important). Why should we question the word of scientists, after all? So, us women do not like sex? Really? Today we know that without stimulating our friend the clitoris, our sex life would be very sad. In reality, the female orgasm is almost entirely clitoral. There, I said it! And there's one more important thing to carve in stone: arousal and our sexual needs are not tied to gender. There is not one way to experience sexuality. The spectrum of possibilities is much broader than we are told. It's like ice cream. There are many flavors other than chocolate and vanilla. There's also caramel,

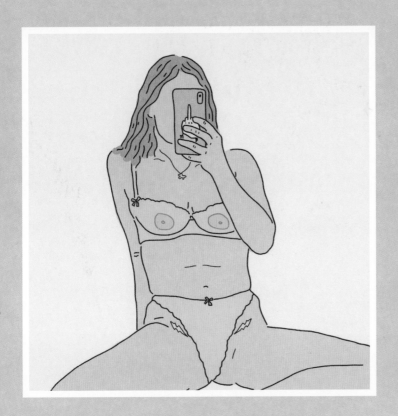

strawberry, chocolate chip, coconut, and many others. There are no rules. The important thing is to listen and learn by getting to know yourself.

#WHOKNOWSYOUBETTERTHANYOU
#FALSETHEORIES   #NORULES
#LISTENTOYOURSELF

Your pleasure is essential,
not secondary to that of others.

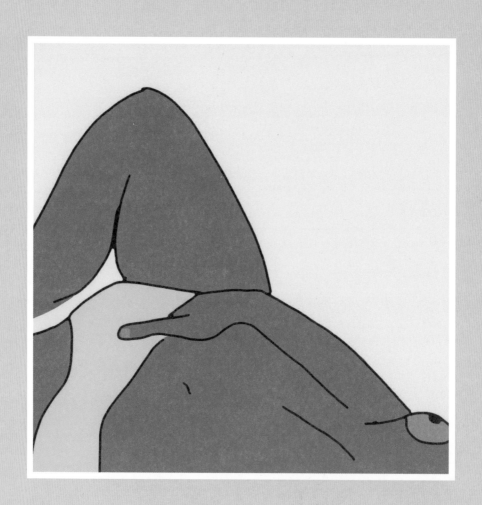

MASTURBATION: NO INHIBITIONS

Masturbation is good for your body, spirit, and health, and there are no downsides. Yes, even women and people with vulvas have a right to do it without hiding or feeling guilty.

For too long, we were made to believe that this pleasure was reserved for men. In the nineteenth century, female arousal was considered "abnormal" or even "dangerous." One of the many ways women were prevented from touching themselves was by pouring acid on their clitoris or removing it! This practice continues to this day in some parts of the world.

Let's not joke around. Us women must be able to masturbate in peace and in many different ways. It's true, there are many techniques and methods for giving ourselves pleasure, exploring, and coming into contact with our senses to get to know ourselves better. So let's give it a chance! But let's not forget that female pleasure is still a huge taboo; to talk about it without shame, we had to fight—and still do.

So c'mon, don't waste time, take a moment for yourself for a solo pleasure session. You won't regret it.

#SOLOPLEASURE
#DATEWITHMYSELF

Touching yourself and fostering positive energy is important . . . in this world of bad vibes.

"WHAT DO YOU LIKE?"

When you move on to having sex with other people, communication is fundamental. However, we aren't used to talking about what we like, perhaps because we are shy or lazy or simply don't think about it. But a relationship is a two-way street (or three . . . or why not more?). And even if it's a fling from Tinder, listening to others is extremely important. We all have different preferences, in life as well as in sex. Of course, sometimes we don't know exactly what we like. Perhaps it's easier for those who are more aware of their sexuality. Each experience is different and has its variables to consider. Most importantly, don't ever forget that the desire to have sex must be reciprocal. Learning to say what we want and knowing what the other likes helps make the experience much more enjoyable. So, what do you like? It's a simple question, but it's still a sensitive issue. We should all ask ourselves this question so that we get to know ourselves and our partners better, set limits, and reach maximum pleasure.

#TELLMEWHATYOULIKE   #SEX
#BETTERCOMMUNICATIONBETTERSEX

What do I like, and what do you like?
That is the question.

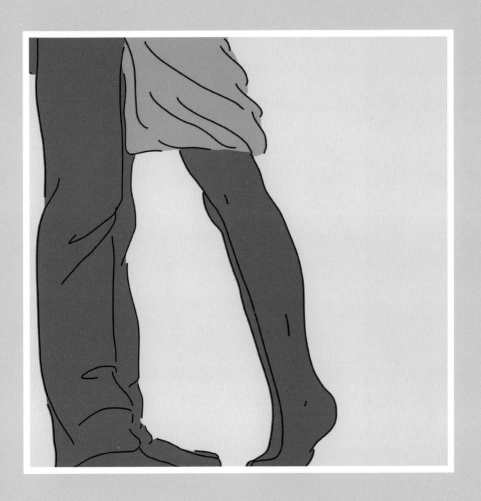

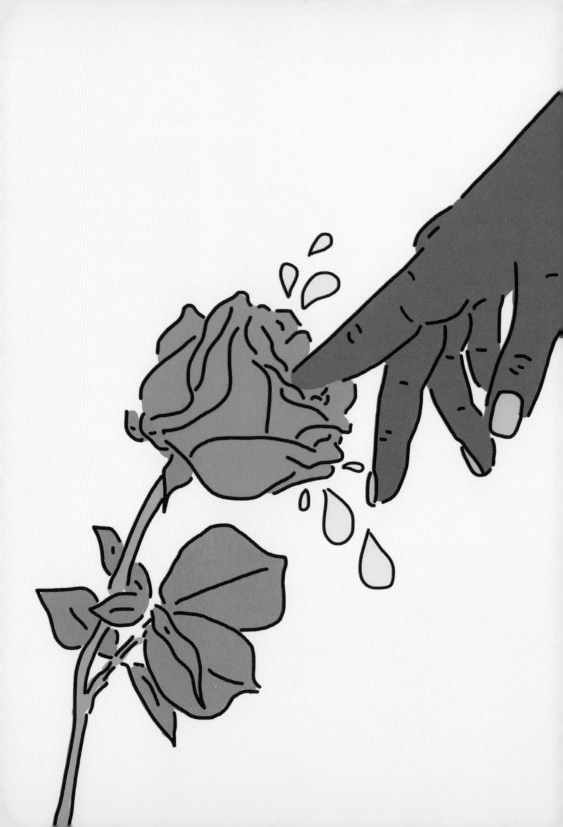

ORGASMS: "OH, YEAH, RIGHT THERE!"

The orgasm. A little pleasure we can't do without! But it's not an end in itself; you can have fun even without it. And it should never become a source of stress! "Chacun fait-fait-fait c'qui lui plait-plait-plait" ("Everyone does-does-does what they want-want-want," cit. Chagrin d'amour)!!! Oops, sorry. We were saying . . . ?

Orgasms are good for you. They release hormones and make you feel euphoric! You can achieve it on your own or with another. The annoying thing is that we are always told that male orgasm is easy to achieve, whereas female orgasm is a luxury, often called "complicated" or considered difficult to achieve. But now we know that the pleasure organ is the clitoris, and you can have an orgasm in just a few seconds and multiple times. So, if it doesn't always happen, don't panic. Some advice: if you've never had one, go out right now and buy a vibrator. It'll be hard to fail. And when you reach the top, you'll feel amazing!

#HAPPINESSHORMONES

#ALONEORTOGETHER

Whether you achieve it or not is not the point; but when you do, it'll be so good.

CENSORING FEMALE SEXUAL APPETITES

"Slut shaming" implies that a woman's enjoyment of sex is a serious and damaging attitude, making her a slut. Society perpetuates and normalizes the idea that men are naturally sexual beings, whereas women's sexuality is of little or no importance. Sex is something that women receive passively, without consent. Therefore, when women show desire and sexuality, it seems crazy. But cis men don't have a monopoly over sexual appetite! Why shouldn't women have the right to talk about sex or masturbation? We have the right to enjoy things as we please, without limits on who or how. In other words, let's do what we want. In our society, which is confusing and contradictory, everyone should be free to make their own choices, in all areas. And our value has nothing to do with the number of sexual partners we have. Period. Mic drop.

#FREEDOM   #WHATDOYOUKNOW
#PROUDTOBEASLUT

Let's stop humiliating women who appreciate sex.

MANEATER

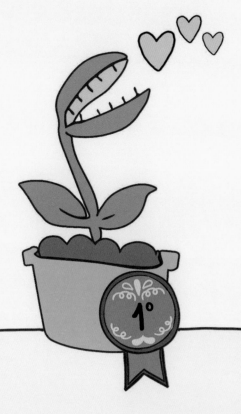

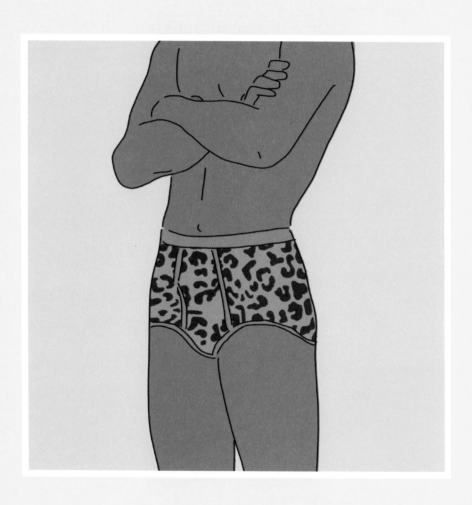

THE FAN OF POSSIBILITIES

In the modern world, we love boxes and putting people, along with their sexual orientation, gender, and identity, in them. But it's not always possible to see yourself in one of these predetermined boxes. The range of possibilities is much broader than you can imagine. We have sexual preferences that are sometimes very clear and sometimes not yet well defined. No pressure. It could take some time to understand them. The important thing is developing as an individual. Of course, today this is a much discussed and debated topic that brings out numerous conflicts, on a personal level, among family, and within society. To me, it's important to listen and not let yourself be too influenced by social pressure. We would risk not listening to how we feel about so-called "normality." If you are afraid of being yourself, as many of us are, it's never too late to change your mind. When you feel it, do not hesitate: speak up and reclaim who you are.

#LONGLIVESINCERITY

#SEXUALITYISASPECTRUM

Sexual orientation is not a problem to be solved.

CONSENT OVER EVERYTHING

Unfortunately, we must continue to repeat this. Because, for many, "consent" is still a bit of an obscure concept. So, let's clear it up:

Consent has nothing to do with the length of your skirt. It's not about interpreting signs. Only one word means yes, and that's "yes." Everything else, from "I don't know" to "No," does not mean "Maybe" or "Go ahead and try." It means "No."

We must teach this imperative value to children and teach them to respect when someone says "No."

When we talk about sexual relations, thinking that explicit consent ruins the atmosphere is just plain idiocy . . . and the only ones who believe this are those who truly don't care about consent.

As if that weren't enough, society also struggles to accept a woman who says "Yes." Because, in truth, she would do well to censor herself. But desire is not a male privilege. We all have the right to desire, and therefore we all have the right to refuse what we don't desire.

#NOMEANSNO   #ANEXPLICITYES
#CONSENTISSEXY

"No" means *no*, and if it's not an explicit "Yes," it also means *no*.

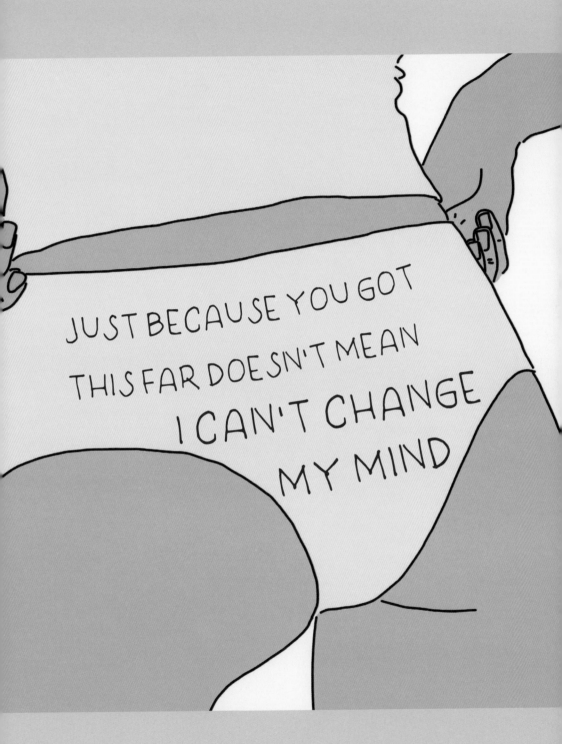

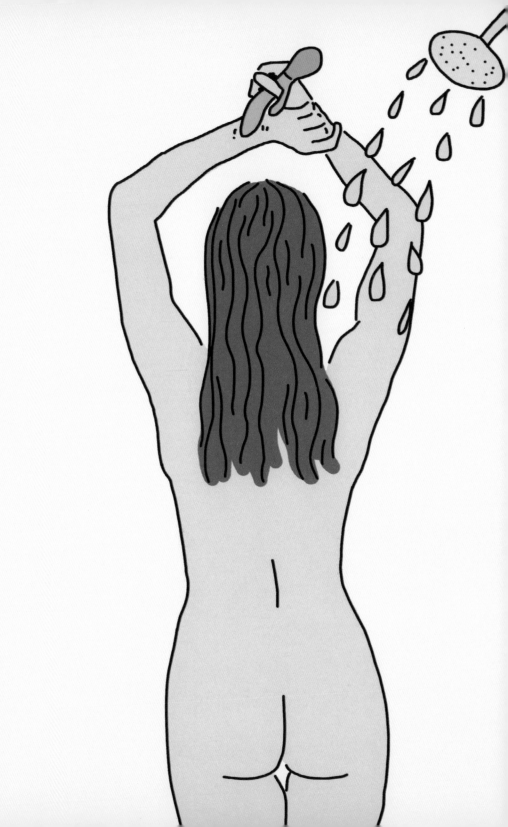

SPOIL YOURSELF WITH SEX TOYS

What a great invention, sex toys! Love, attention, pleasure: we deserve it all. When I was a girl, I thought they were only for strange, obsessed adults. I had this image of a hidden shop you wouldn't dare venture into for fear you'd cross eyes with a man in a trench coat who followed you, snickering as he exposed himself. I admit, it must have been a nightmare I had. Today, sex shops are more like any retail storefront than a horror-themed escape room. Now it's "the magical world of sex toys," an enchanted place for adults. There's something for everyone. Brands offer more and more products for all variety of pleasures.

Buying them and talking about them have become much less taboo. If you still haven't gotten a sex toy, I suggest you do so immediately. Trust me, a vibrator will change your life!

#SEXTOYSFORALL   #VIBRATORPOWER

#UNLIMITEDBUDGETSEXTOYS

Adults can have toys, too!

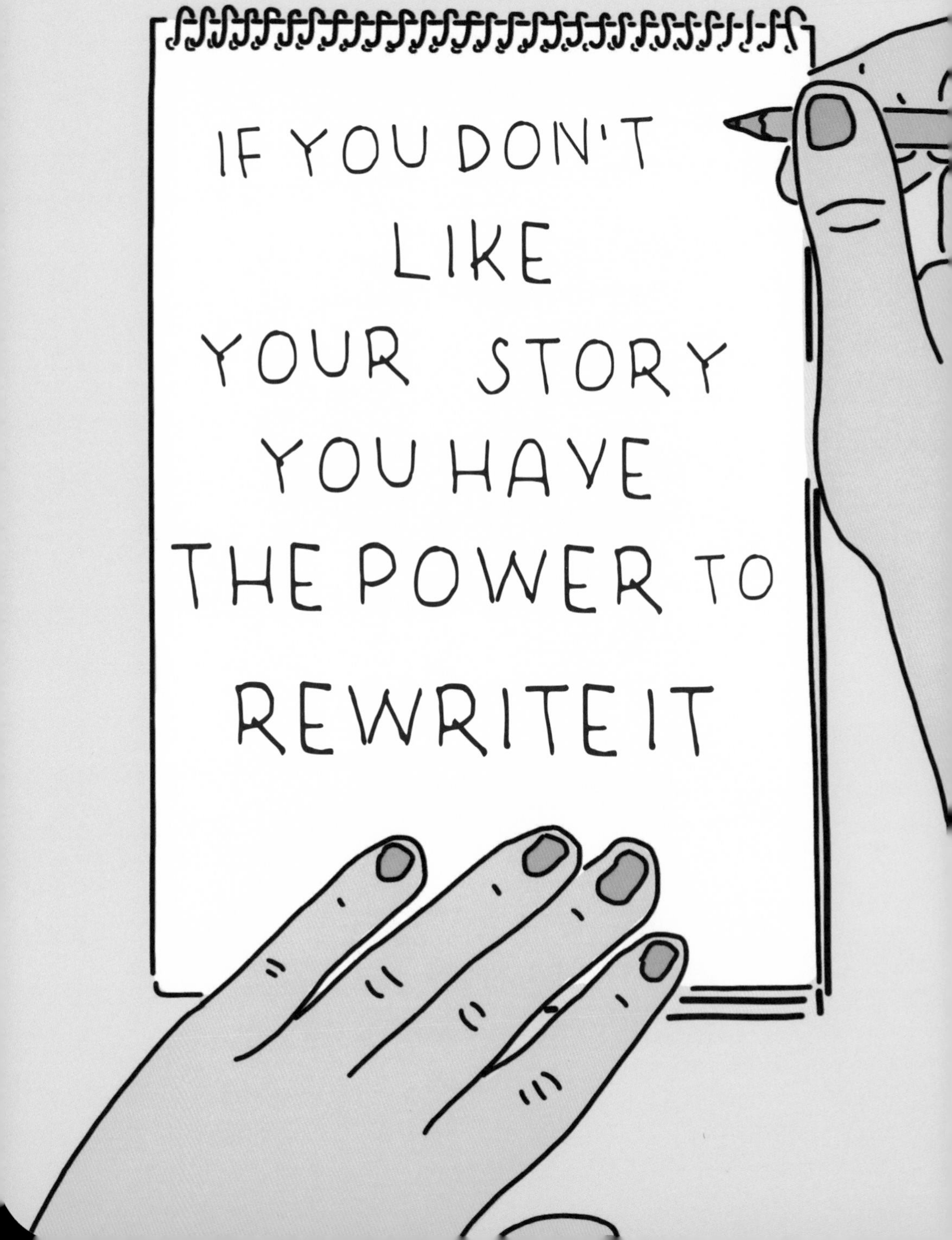

IF YOU DON'T
LIKE
YOUR STORY
YOU HAVE
THE POWER TO
REWRITE IT

· · · · ·

Chapter 4

The Art of Real Change

· · · · ·

We can go on with our heads down, without thinking about our states of mind or the things that hurt us, telling ourselves we will deal with them later. Or we can learn to understand ourselves. Look yourself in the eye and get in touch with your inner self. Once we start to really listen and look at the beautiful things around us—like trees at a nearby park—we can then breathe deeply and take a step toward inner peace.

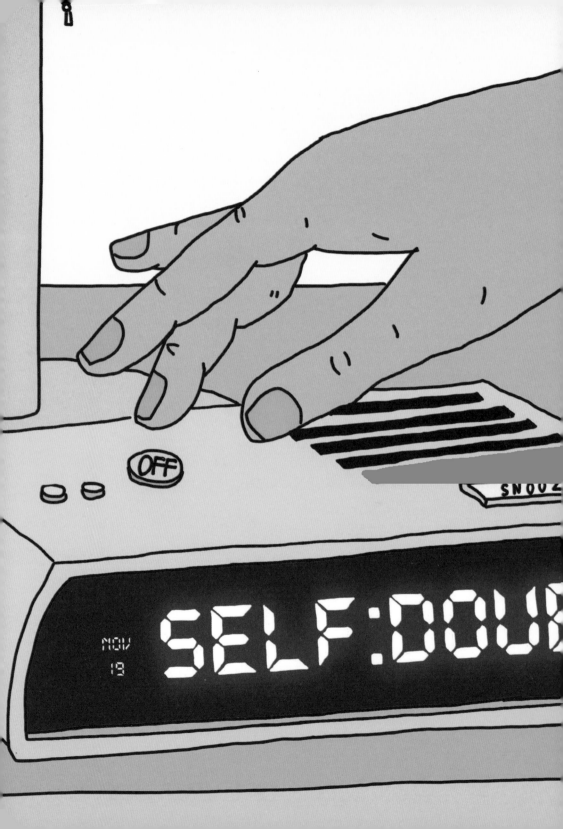

MIND VS. SPIRIT

The mind and spirit: a very important topic on the road to self-acceptance. In simple terms, the mind is the sort of scary little voice we often hear that doesn't always help us make the right decision. It's a confusing mix of ideas that we started storing in our heads since childhood. A potpourri of education, morals, experiences, and emotions that weighs us down. "I don't know what I want to do. Eat this. Don't eat that. Exercise! Will I ever manage to achieve something in life?"

Spirit, on the other hand, is much lighter. It allows us to see things as they are and accept them without judgment. "I am who I am and I don't need to become someone else. Go away, scary little voice in my head!"

See the difference? Well, it's easy to say; but when we start to get into touch with ourselves and block out all the noise, we take a huge step toward personal growth.

#MENTALHEALTH   #INNERPEACE
#INTOUCHWITHMYSELF

Don't be your own obstacle.

EMBRACING EMOTIONS

"She's hysterical!" "Is she on her period, or what?" These comments are "normal" observations when a woman gets angry. And then, "Crying is weak," especially if you are a man. In the binary system, it is a totally shameful behavior for males. Hmpf! The result? Wherever you are on the spectrum of gender and sexuality, we are all condemned to evade our emotions and imprison this natural energy that will only eventually become trauma, or worse.

- (Inner voice): "Laetitia, stay calm. . . ."
- "But it's making me so angry!"
- "Yes, but you are a woman. You can't get angry; you must be kind, docile, calm, and pleasant."
- "Oh, shut up, f*****!"

Oops! Well, anyway. . . . Our emotions are a natural phenomenon; but when they come from our mind, that pesky little voice that often plays terrible jokes on us, we try to control them. Denying or suffocating them is not a healthy solution, because it prevents us from understanding them. And the idea is to learn to understand them without judgment.

#DIRTYTRICKSOFEMOTIONS

#OBSERVINGEMOTIONS   #ACCEPTINGEMOTIONS

**Paying attention to our emotions
is the secret to accepting them.**

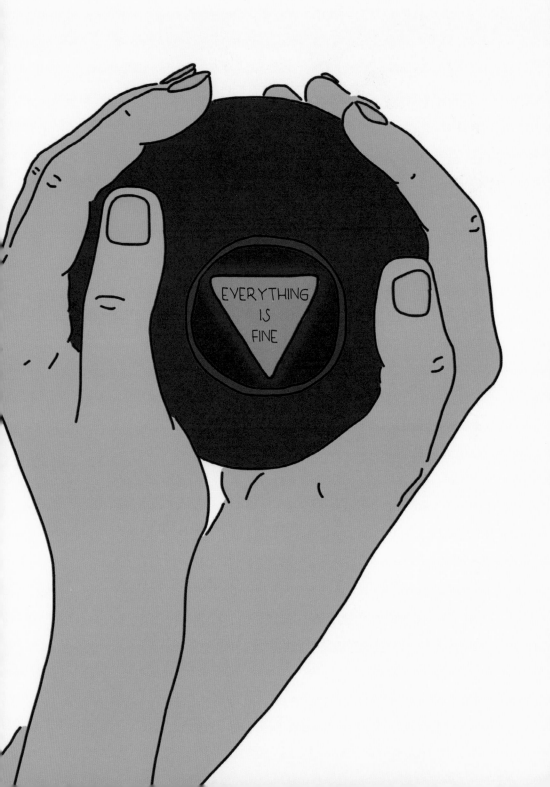

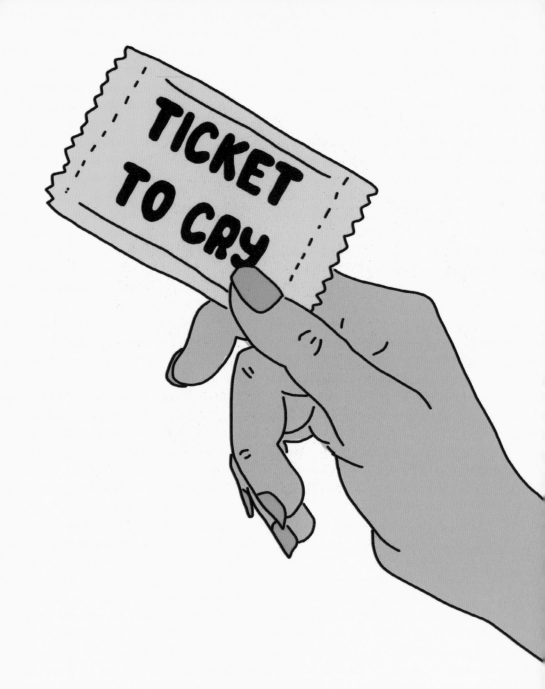

IT'S OKAY TO CRY

Apparently, we are the only creatures that cry. Crazy, huh? Unfortunately, in a lot of ways the older we get, the more difficult life becomes. The shift from childhood to adulthood is hard, a change that many of us do not want to make because the world of adults seems like a mess with all its obligations and responsibilities. Who doesn't want to cry every once in a while? The myth of always needing to be strong is a fantasy! We are often told as children, especially boys, to "Be strong," or "Don't cry, it's nothing," even when it's serious to us. But crying is okay! We are all vulnerable beings, and as children we cry, no matter our gender.

If we accept this vulnerability, we realize that it is a strength and that we should not have to hide it. Tears also stimulate "happiness hormones." Crying has many benefits. It reduces stress, makes us realize that something doesn't work for us, and socially is a way to ask for help. In other words, crying is cool and healthy. Why shouldn't you?

#ITSOKTOCRY   #HAPPINESSHORMONES
#CRYINGISFREEING

A little, a lot, sometimes . . . let yourself go, let your emotions flow!

SELF-CARE: MAKE IT A PRIORITY

Taking care of and not neglecting yourself seems logical, no? But do we really take care of ourselves? We all have our doses of delusions, terrible and toxic relationships, and disastrous meetings. And we tell ourselves "This is shit!" But we continue to push onward until we are out of breath. We are social animals, and we need interaction with others. We believe we have to be "likable" at all costs . . . and we forget to set boundaries. We let ourselves go to systematic comparison, as if life were a competition. We spend our free time on social media, scrolling and examining other people's success stories. We get the impression that everyone has a wonderful life except us. We dream of becoming someone who doesn't match who we truly are. We tend to treat ourselves poorly. There is a middle ground, a balance between oneself and the other. And if we are kind to others, we should be kind to ourselves too! We can do many small things to reclaim our personal time and energy. Luckily, our bodies will tell us when we are neglecting them or when we are not in harmony with ourselves. It is a matter of energy! Let's listen without forgetting that "Your life is yours, and no one else lives it!"

#OBSERVEYOURSELF   #SELFCARE
#YOURWELLBEINGMATTERS   #ITSWORTHIT
#RESPECTYOURNEEDS

Taking care of yourself shouldn't be a luxury.

IT'S OKAY TO PUT YOURSELF FIRST AT TIMES. DON'T FEEL GUILTY FOR DOING WHAT'S RIGHT FOR YOU

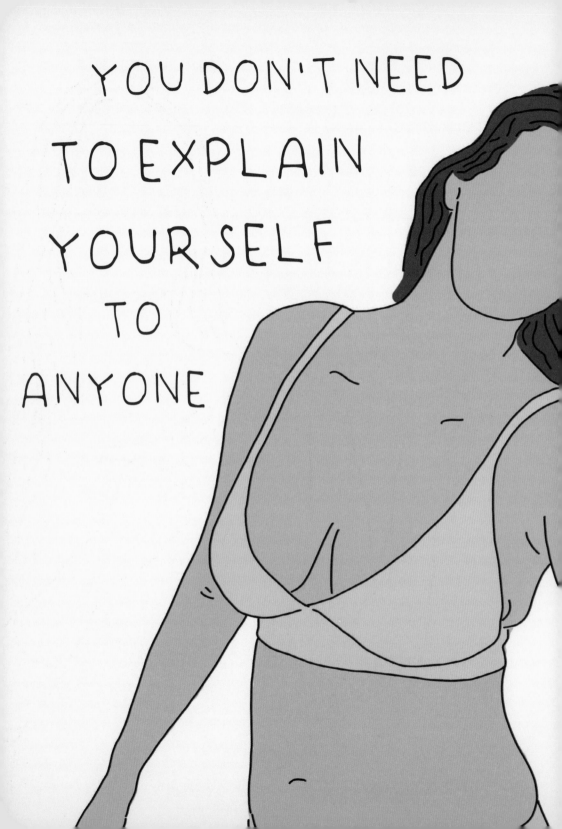

KNOW HOW TO SAY NO

For a long time, I struggled to say no. Perhaps it is because I didn't want to be unpleasant or feared ruining the image someone had of me. And in the world we live in, we always have the impression that we must be present, hyper-productive . . . always running! But we must not let others consume our energy, or they may walk all over us. Some people are not aware (or choose not to be aware) of other people's boundaries. They don't seem to understand that relationships are not a one-way street, demanding energy and attention without giving any in return. It takes time and perspective to understand that these types of relationships are not healthy and cannot continue as they are. Usually, we are at the edge of a nervous breakdown when we finally throw out a very shy and quiet "No," but inside it's a loud cry. We can't take it anymore. Then "No" becomes more natural and makes us feel better.

This NO must be heard and understood, and that's true for all unpleasant situations or simply things we don't have the energy for.

#SETBOUNDARIES   #YOUCANSAYNO
#NOTHANKS   #YESCANMEANNO

If it's not what you are looking for or what you need, if it hurts you, the answer is "No." There's no need to explain. "No" is a complete sentence.

FOOD: FRIEND, NOT FOE

Unfortunately, many of us have complicated relationships with food. Let's be clear: the patriarchy has been in this realm as well, and it has left its mark, especially on women . . . how strange. You don't believe me? So, then, where does diet culture come from? A woman must be thin, but not too thin, and she must watch her figure and weight. While men dig in, we must nibble! At least figuratively. Are you following me? When it's not people around us repeating "Eat less or you'll gain weight," or "Eat more, you're too thin," it's our own minds and the internalized misogyny that put pressure on us. We blame ourselves if we eat what we want. Sometimes we want junk food; so what? When we are struggling and down, we look for comfort in food. But since we place too much importance on numbers—age, weight, size, inches—it doesn't take much to develop a love-hate relationship with food.

#LIFESPLEASURES

#EATWHATYOUWANT

#DONTEXPLAINYOURFOOD

Enjoy eating and the foods you love!

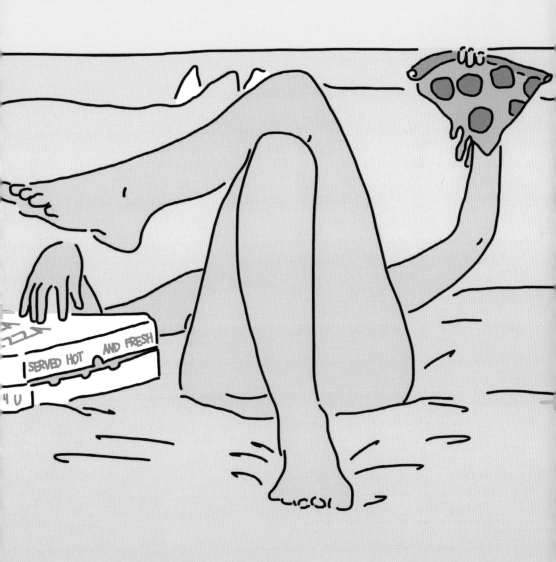

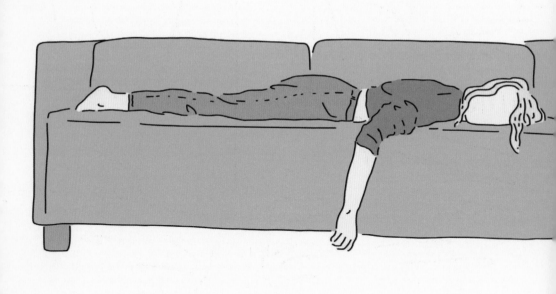

MOTIVATION UNDER PRESSURE (NOTHING TO PROVE)

Just thinking about motivation makes me tired ;-). It takes a large amount of energy to keep motivation high. When you are a woman, you need it first thing in the morning! Taking a shower, putting on makeup, doing your hair: it takes the better part of an hour. Three, if you're a true perfectionist!

I learned to reevaluate my motivation because, as a woman in the world we live in, I always have something more to prove. As if women don't deserve the jobs and duties they have, or stole them from men who obviously deserved it more. It's all a patriarchal invention, obviously. Women demonstrate their abilities every day in all tasks, and we are just as good as men. And besides, what's with this rush to be productive? You aren't less important if you aren't busy. Sometimes it's better to stop for two minutes or even to refuse an offer. And there's no need to question our value because we decide to take a break!

#NOTHINGTOPROVE

#LOWMOTIVATION

#STOPEXCESSIVEPRODUCTIVITY

Our worth isn't measured with productivity.

YOUR HEART BEATS FOR YOU

When we think of Love with a capital L, we often think of romcom movies, cheesy songs, and couples. Now I don't want to say that couple love doesn't exist, but sometimes we confuse it with something else. Sometimes, this leads to unhealthy relationships that we can't get out of, perhaps because we think we don't deserve better. So here we are at the importance of Self-love with a capital S! It might sound selfish, and often we try to push it away! But we must repeat it: YOU are your first love!

Loving ourselves is a strength that shouldn't be underestimated! It means making decisions for ourselves, no exceptions. My future self will thank me for saying "No" or "Bye-bye" to situations and people who aren't good for me.

Being aware of our value is a shield against outside attacks. When we love ourselves, there's no space for confusion. Our spirit is solid, unmoving. It doesn't judge us.

#LOVEEVERYWHERE   **#LOVEYOURSELF**
#YOUAREYOURFIRSTLOVE

Listen up! If you think you are not "enough,"
who would think otherwise? You are your first love!
So treat yourself right, with respect
and no compromises.

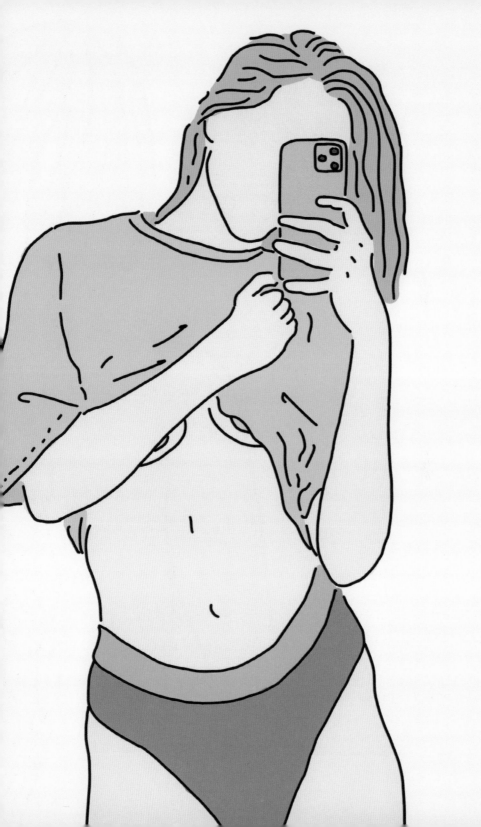

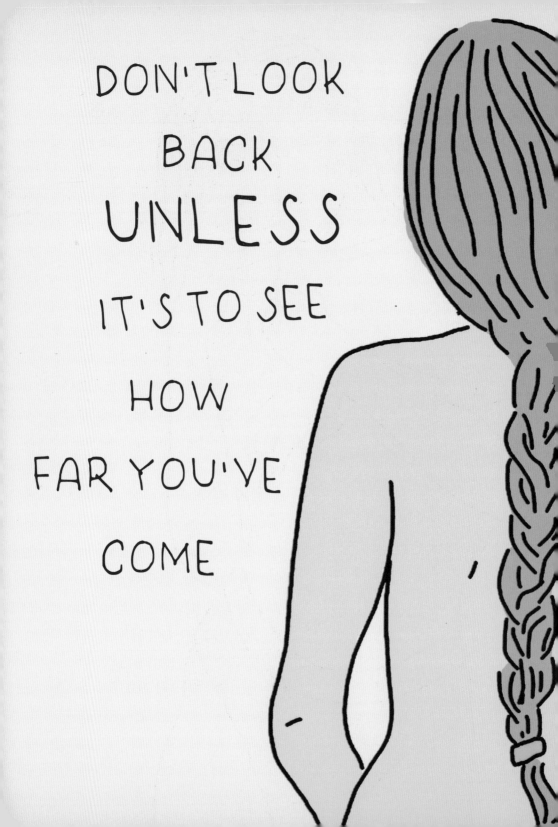

THE ROAD TO SELF-ACCEPTANCE

Self-acceptance is the foundation of our lives. And the sooner you start, the sooner you can find balance. Between the confusion in our heads and that in the environment around us, there's quite a lot of work to go around! Instead of teaching ourselves social success and competition, wouldn't it be better to encourage ourselves to discover and celebrate ourselves in our entirety, to understand and appreciate our unique traits? Of course, this would ruin the career of some plastic surgeons who would be forced to find a new job.

Down with our physical, psychological, and mental standards! Every person is unique, and when we can be honest with ourselves and recognize our strengths and weaknesses, we foster a very positive attitude toward ourselves. Accepting ourselves helps us figure out what we like and what we don't, and this is crucial: it gives us the possibility of developing and improving our lives. Accepting ourselves is a process and can take time, but it is truly worth starting.

#LEARNTOLOVEYOURSELF

#ACCEPTYOURSELFASYOUARE

#KNOWYOURSELFTOPROTECTYOURSELF

This is something we all need!

IN THE CROSSFIRE OF JUDGMENT

Women are constantly being judged and, believe me, it's not a walk in the park. We are bombarded by expectations of how we should be and how we should act. We must have boobs, and big ones, but, please, not too big! And we have to wear heels . . . because we need to be tall and slender! But don't be taller than your partner; it would dishonor his virility. A woman must have curves; she can't look like a twig, but she shouldn't be fat! Start dieting! And be natural! Everything must be orderly, always. It's just one judgment after another, one contradiction after another. It starts at the most vulnerable age and continues into the world of working, making it increasingly hard to please when trying to get a job. We are judged on things like social skills, knowledge, morals, and appearance. We constantly face criticism and judgment. . . .

Stop.

Cancel everything. Press on and do whatever you want.

#EASYTOJUDGE

#KEEPYOURJUDGMENTTOYOURSELF

#ITSHARDBEINGAWOMAN

It's not simple being a woman in a world that is quick to judge. We must erect shields of self-love and indifference.

WOMEN DON'T OWE YOU S**T

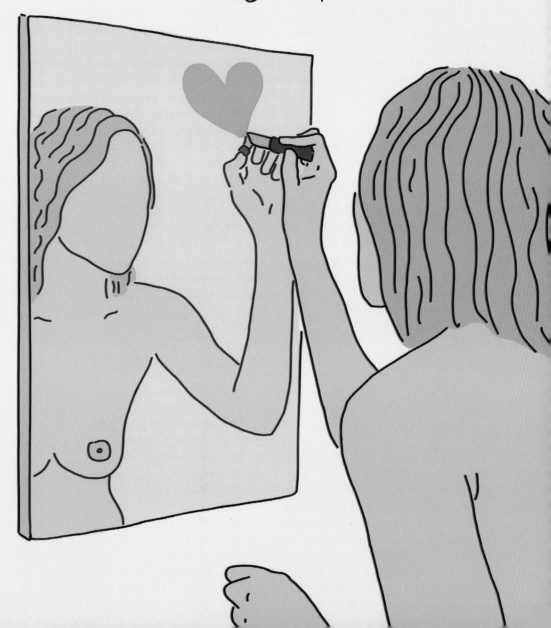

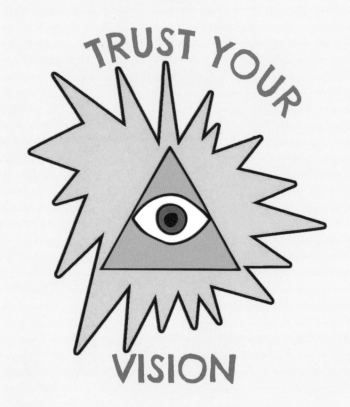

CREATIVITY: TRUST YOUR VISION

We can all be creative and intuitive. We must trust ourselves and stop thinking we are not enough. We all have something to say. The important thing is to be original. You can admire, but avoid copying! We have all done it because we've doubted our own abilities. But making a mistake is not a crime. You can start over again.

Creativity is a source of well-being because it frees us. It can also provoke suffering, but it is mostly good for liberation. Creativity requires concentration, but these days it is difficult to avoid being absorbed by our phones or computers and to not overanalyze what happens on social media for fear of missing out on something. We tend to go toward the noise and confusion, but creativity needs inner space. It feeds off our experiences, our ability to look around us, contemplate, and explore.

If we then add a good dose of hard work, concentration, and liberation, we find that our creativity can be fun and unlimited.

#INFINITECREATIVITY

#CREATIVEINTELLIGENCE

Open your heart, and your creativity will be endless.

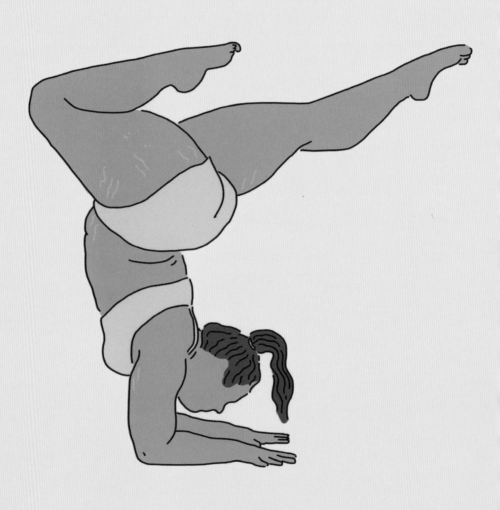

Chapter 5

· · · · ·

Healthy, Ill, or Just Different?

· · · · ·

Health is wealth. The old proverb is still true today.
But when it comes to this, we aren't all the same.
Our anatomical, hormonal, genetic, and social differences
come into play. And let's be clear, illnesses that primarily affect
women have long been pushed aside. What's more is that we should
ask ourselves whether something is actually an illness, or if our
imposed standards just make us feel like something is an "illness"
when it's actually just "different."

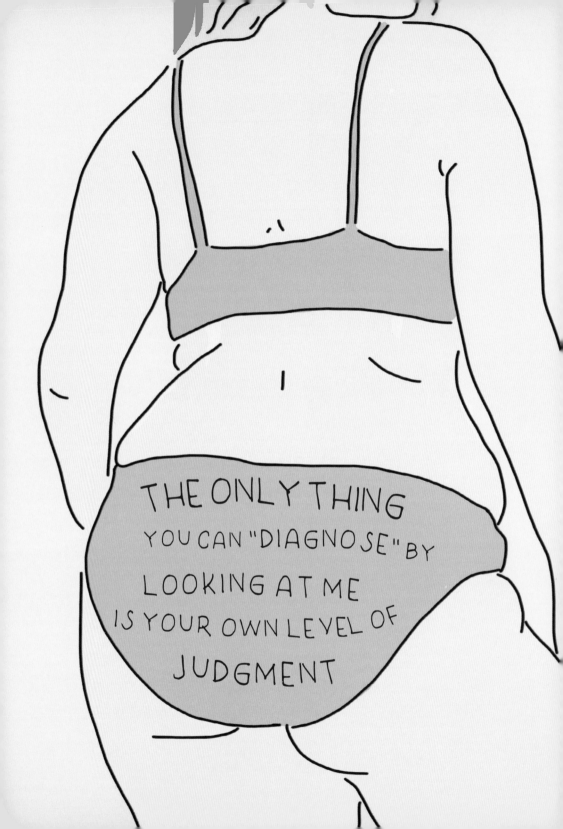

HEALTH IS INVISIBLE

Medicine and research have come a long way and continue moving forward every day. This is especially true for the health concerns of men because, as we've said, we live in a patriarchal society. Men have monopolized the medical world, giving priority to their needs and pushing those of women to the wayside.

In the name of health, there are standards that determine what appearance we should have. But this isn't necessarily tied to our health. The shell doesn't always reveal what's going on inside the body. "Looking sick" is an invention, and there are people who struggle with invisible illnesses (or spread them, perhaps unaware), whereas, for example, being fat doesn't automatically indicate respiratory problems. Enough with these clichés. Haven't you ever heard that appearances can be deceptive?

#REFLECT   #LISTEN
#APPEARANCESAREDECEIVING

Someone's appearance doesn't necessarily reflect their health.

ENDOMETRIOSIS: IT'S NOT A TREND, IT'S AN ILLNESS

D o you get painful cramps that make you want to vomit? I know something about that. It started little by little . . . increasingly violent cramps with episodes that made me want to bang my head against a wall. The arrival of my period became a nightmare. Stabbing pain in my back and stomach . . . it was a horrific scene that would last until I puked. Your period is never a pleasant time, but problems like this are too much. So I did my own research and found out that there is a little-known gynecological illness called endometriosis, which affects **one out of every ten women**. After verifying that I had the symptoms, I assumed that I had it. I tried to get a diagnosis, but finding a doctor who would give me formal confirmation was a battle. One gynecologist even laughed in my face, saying that endometriosis was just the latest trend. It was one of those moments in which I asked myself, "Am I just being weak and wimpy?"

But know this: if you have cramps that make you writhe in pain, first, it is not the latest trend, and second, it is not acceptable! Don't waste time; go see an endometriosis specialist. And rest assured, there are treatments that can alleviate and stabilize the pain. It can also be kept in check with diet. Personally, ever since I started exercising regularly, the pain has been much less intense, and episodes are rare. I am a new person! But the strange thing is that this illness—benign but very painful—is still so misunderstood!

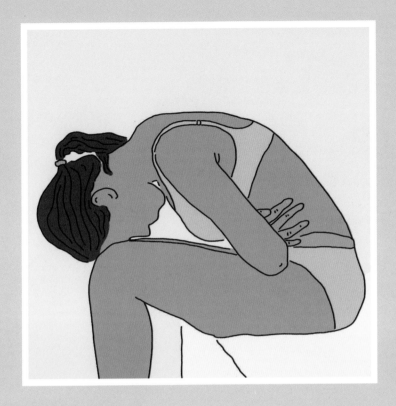

It's fundamental that women conduct medical research, so that illnesses that affect us are not neglected but actively studied!

#FEMALEILLNESSES

#ANSWERFORENDOMETRIOSIS

#STOPSUFFERINGINSILENCE

Are we supposed to suffer in silence just because we live in a patriarchal world?

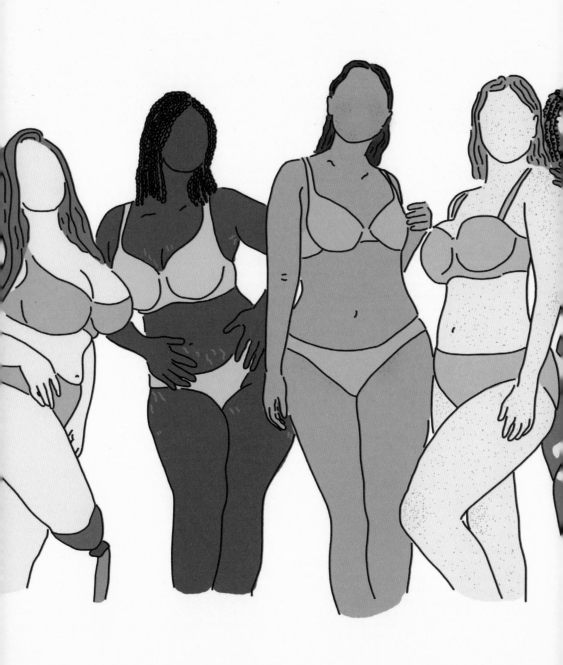

ILLNESS AND DISABILITY: INCLUSIVITY POWERS "BODY POSITIVITY"

It's not easy to live with "physical deformities" in a society that is founded on the cult of perfection and performance. That's why inclusion is fundamental. People with illnesses and disabilities have to live with their differences and learn to tolerate the sometimes-mocking looks of others. It is a daily battle. But with social media, we have seen a community of people emerge and shine a light on their differences and even provide resources. They fearlessly show their scars, prosthetics, medical aid, or wheelchairs to foster awareness. These activists teach us a valuable lesson about self-acceptance and give us an important reminder that inclusion is beautiful! Sharing positive ideas on this topic—through media, art, and fashion—is so important to help support and to question our understanding of health. We all deserve to be seen, represented, and accepted and to enjoy the capabilities of our bodies.

#ACCEPTINGYOURDIFFERENCES

#RAREBEAUTY   #INCLUSIONISPOWERFUL

The visible difference: an original and powerful mark.

FEMALE TUMORS: UNDERSTANDING AND PREVENTING THEM!

Cancer is the disease of the century! And we still have not found a definitive cure or preventative measure. There is research, but there are still many unanswered questions, and we still don't know what exactly happens in an afflicted body. It would seem that we all have some cancerous cells that can develop or not. That's why regular check-ups are so important. Breast tumors affect a large number of women. Eight out of ten cases occur past fifty years of age, but we shouldn't assume it's something that only happens to others. We must remain vigilant! Likewise, it's important at every age to have regular Pap tests and avoid getting human papillomavirus (HPV), which can highly increase the risk of a cervical tumor. Now women can get vaccinated against HPV, so inform yourself! I think that stress and frustration, if ignored or neglected, can create favorable conditions for the formation of certain illnesses. That's another reason why self-acceptance is so important.

#IGETREGULARPAPS   #PAPTEST
#CANCER   #GETINFORMED
#PAYATTENTIONTOHEALTH

Get checked regularly to help protect your health!

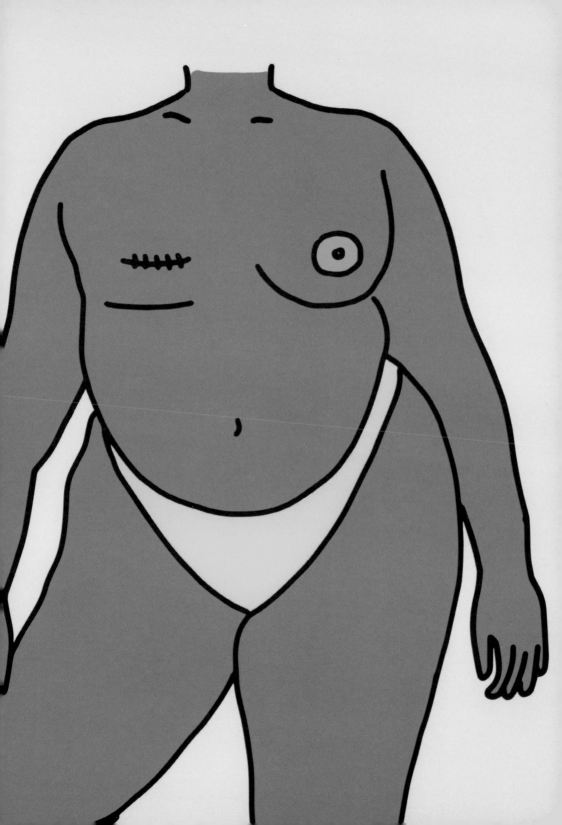

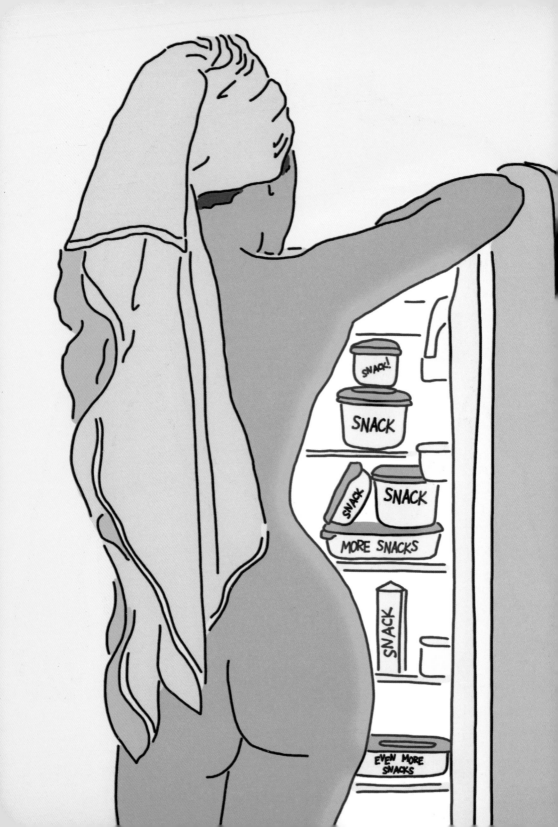

BULIMIA OR UNCONTROLLED FEEDING

Bulimia is an eating disorder characterized by a pathological relationship with food that manifests through repeated and persistent binge eating (to the point of feeling sick). It is often connected to unresolved psychological disorders. It mainly affects young women and girls between the ages of eleven and twenty, but it often persists because healing is a long process, and the disorder is often confronted and overcome many years later. Freeing yourself of the pain that comes with it from a young age is difficult. We are born with a certain personality, but are generally poorly educated on self-acceptance and self-worth, even if many parents don't have ill intentions. Then there's school, social pressure, and the absurdities of the world—we must go through it all to rediscover ourselves as we were, as our pure self, with the aspects of our character and without the wounds that have accumulated.

#OVERCOMINGBULIMIA
#BULIMIA   #FILLINGAVOID

Your body does not determine your value.

ANOREXIA: ALWAYS FEELING OVERWEIGHT

Anorexia is another dangerous eating disorder that can seriously weaken the body, causing various symptoms, like the absence of menstruation, and can even in extreme cases lead to death. Anorexia is more prevalent in women. It is the result of such intense pressure regarding physical appearance that some adolescents and fragile young women grow up with a phobia of getting fat. They see themselves as overweight. They have a warped perception of their image. At first they feel good, happy to lose weight; but little by little they start to lose faith in themselves, which can lead to depression. Experts don't exactly know where it comes from, but there is a serious problem with education on this topic that must be remedied immediately. Listening to our children and taking active steps aimed at improving their well-being are fundamental.

#OVERCOMINGANOREXIA   #ANOREXIA
#SELFIMAGE
#YOURIMAGEISNOTYOURWORTH

We must remain vigilant when overcoming eating disorders!

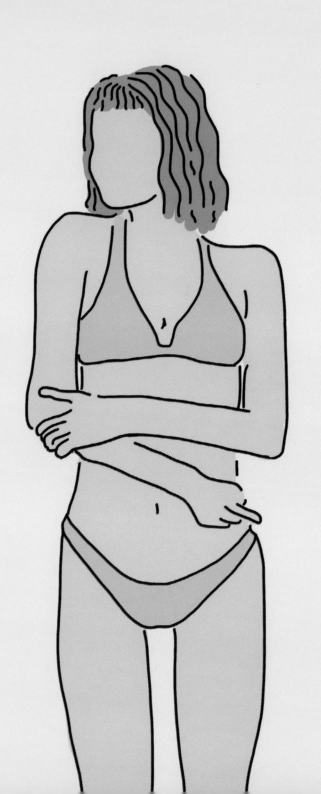

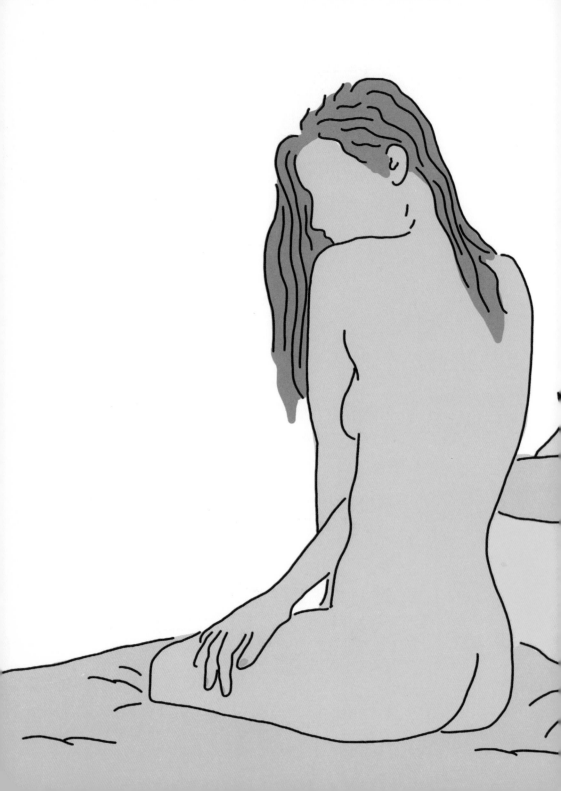

ANORGASMIA: HELP, I CAN'T ORGASM

We can orgasm even in the absence of desire just as we can have desire but not orgasm. This is called anorgasmia. This phenomenon affects more than a quarter of the women in the world. And yet it is a huge taboo. Since society insists that the orgasm is the end goal of sexuality, those who can't orgasm feel "abnormal." It causes a race to orgasm in intimate moments that tends to be rather counterproductive.

There are many causes and degrees of anorgasmia, and they are often tied to mental issues more than physical ones, whether they are known or not. It can be caused by trauma, such as sexual assault, but often it is sparked by factors like lack of self-trust, modesty or fear, education that is too strict, or difficulty accepting your own desires. To overcome mental blocks and embrace pleasure, you must communicate with your partner and know yourself. Pleasure is a spectrum that goes beyond just achieving an orgasm.

#ACCEPTYOURSEXUALITY

#WELCOMEPLEASURE

#ORGASMSARENOTTHEENDGOAL

#PLEASUREDOESNOTEQUALORGASM

The road to pleasure starts with having a sex life that reflects your desires.

UTIs, ENEMY OF THE BLADDER

Urinary tract infections (UTIs) are very common, affecting one out of every two women. It occurs more frequently when first becoming sexually active and after menopause. It is an inflammation of the bladder usually caused by the bacteria Escherichia coli; in simple terms, it's when it burns when you pee. Yes, it can be painful, but it can also be asymptomatic or simply annoying. Usually it is easy to cure, but it must be dealt with. It is often incompetently treated, which can make it much more difficult to cure. Some people develop recurrent UTIs, causing a downward spiral of endless stress and too much medication. Come on, ladies, we must annihilate this problem. Don't listen to anyone who minimizes your pain.

#TALKABOUTUTIS

#GIVEWOMENAVOICE

#DIFFICULTBLADDERS

UTIs are very common. We must talk about it so it doesn't become a taboo!

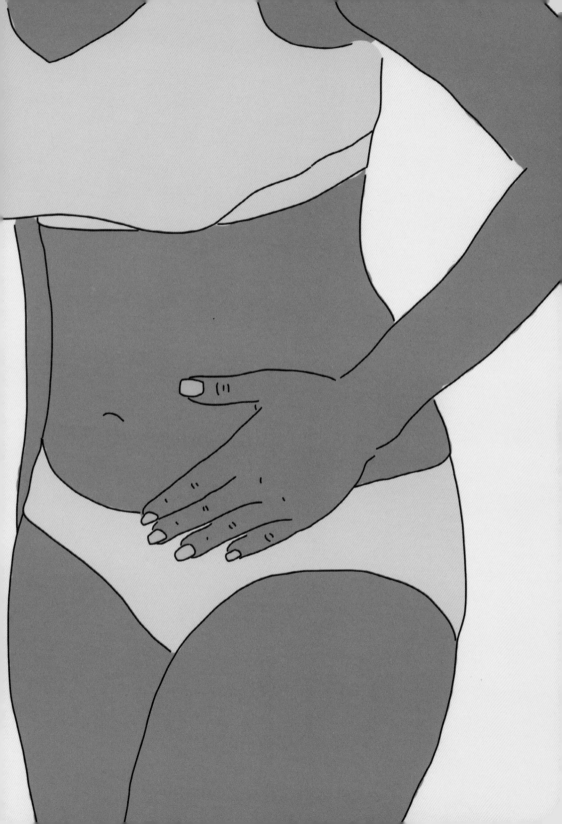

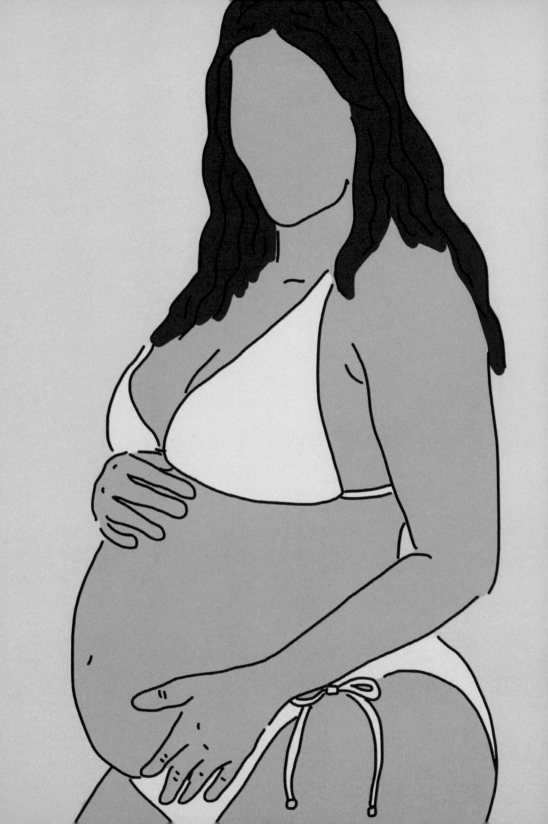

. . . . .

Chapter 6

Reproduction at the Heart of the Patriarchal System

. . . . .

The uterus—and its reproductive abilities—is, like we said, of great interest to men, who wish to impose their own rules on it. But it's a simple fact: the uterus belongs to those who have one! And when we give birth, the question is "To whom does the child belong?" Women birth them, but, in many cultures, they take their father's name. Once again, the patriarchy has left its mark. Science, however, makes it possible for couples who don't fit into the cookie-cutter model of "mother and father" to procreate.

MY BODY,
MY SEXUALITY,
MY MORALS,
MY VOICE,
MY CHOICE

NOTyours

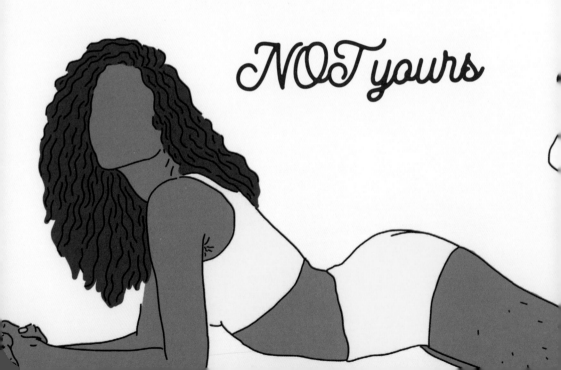

REPRODUCTIVE FREEDOM: IF AND WHEN I WANT

Reproductive freedom is a broad concept that is closely tied to civil, political, and social rights. Put simply, it is about the right to abortion, to education, to contraceptives and all services of reproductive health, as well as equal rights within the family, the right to choose whether you want to marry, and freedom from all discrimination and violence.

Reproductive freedom is one of the most important battles in the fight for the emancipation of women, since it is directly connected to personal dignity and our ability to make decisions about our sexuality.

This fundamental right gives women a certain reproductive autonomy that frees them from unwanted pregnancies. Even though we have been fighting against stereotypes and sexist behavior for over half a century, in many countries social or religious pressure persists that denies women access to these essential rights. It is a continuous fight against the still very male-dominant mentality of our society.

#FEMALEEMANCIPATION
#REPRODUCTIVEAUTONOMY
#REPRODUCTIVEFREEDOM

This fundamental right gives women control over their bodies.

SEXISM IN THE CONTRACEPTIVE INDUSTRY

I don't want to be a killjoy, but thank god for birth control. It prevents us from getting pregnant when we don't want to, and some contraceptive methods can also prevent sexually transmitted diseases! It must not be a taboo. It's called safe sex. Contraception is available in many options: physical, chemical, or surgical. However, the contraceptive industry is sexist. Women undergo constraints and side effects from birth control much more often than men, in addition to the very serious consequences of not using it. The pill, for example, we accept less and less. And for good reason, considering it's not the best for your health. Does it not seem strange that the pill makes your cycle function like clockwork? Personally, when I stopped, bam, pimples and forehead spots! It completely disrupts your hormonal system. It would be nice if men would take it instead of us. Well, then, try it . . . or would that just shift the problem?

#SEXISM   #SIDEEFFECTS
#DOUBLESTANDARDS   #MENTALHEALTH

Women bear the brunt of the unfair burden of contraception.

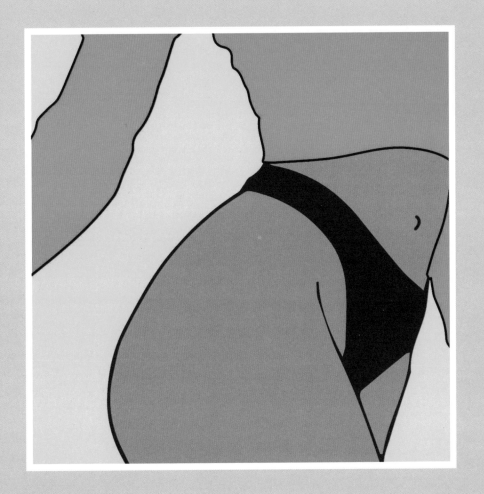

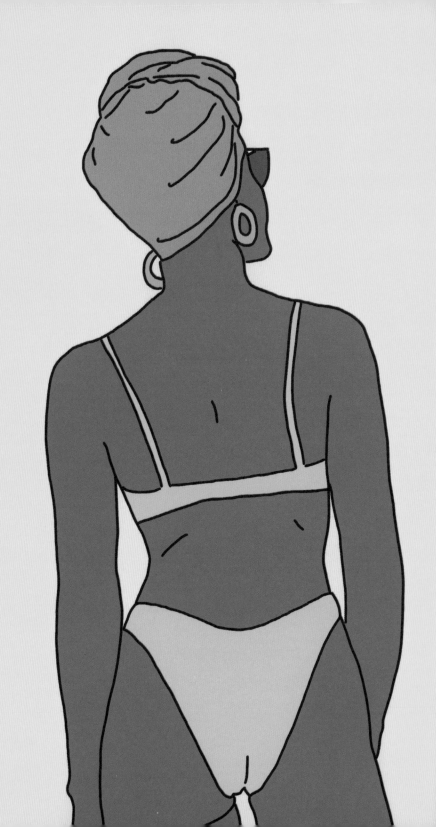

ABORTION: MY BODY, MY DECISION

Abortion is a very serious topic that shouldn't be joked about. But it's really quite simple. We can't give anyone control over our bodies in the name of culture or religion. More importantly, men shouldn't control us. It's been happening for long enough.

Abortion is not taken lightly. They want us to believe that women who abort are irresponsible. Oh, really? Because it's such a fun experience, right? The most scandalous thing should be that sometimes abortions are done secretly in dangerous conditions. Or they are paid for in private clinics when the right to them is denied in public hospitals. That's why it's fundamental that the right to an abortion be recognized and protected, not to increase the number of abortions but to decrease the number of deaths from illegal abortions and the speculation of private offices. Do you see the difference? It must be a personal decision, not political.

#MYBODYMYCHOICE   **#FREEDOM**
#ACCESSFORALL   **#EQUALITY**

Abortion must be safe, legal, and accessible for everyone. Period.

FEMININITY DOES NOT EQUAL MOTHERHOOD

To have a baby, or more than one, wow, that would be nice but also a lot of work. Some women struggle: I've visited a friend who had just given birth and could see how much she was struggling. She wanted me to believe everything was okay, but I could see the stress on her face. I could see the cry for help in her eyes, begging me to take her away, when her mouth says she's never been happier. And then there are women for whom motherhood is child's play: natural, like breathing.

They say that having a child changes your life. It's definitely a very intense journey of initiation, but a woman's self-actualization doesn't necessarily derive from becoming a mother. Femininity and motherhood are often mistakenly intertwined.

In the past, women didn't have the right to decide for themselves, as if they were baby-making machines! But reproducing is not an obligation, and not all women want a child. Furthermore, some can't or have difficulty. Those who don't want to conform to this predominant model are pressured about something that should be a personal decision. Enough.

#BECOMINGAMOTHER

#THERIGHTTONOTBEAMOTHER

#FEMININITYDOESNOTEQUALMOTHERHOOD

You are not obligated to become a mother.

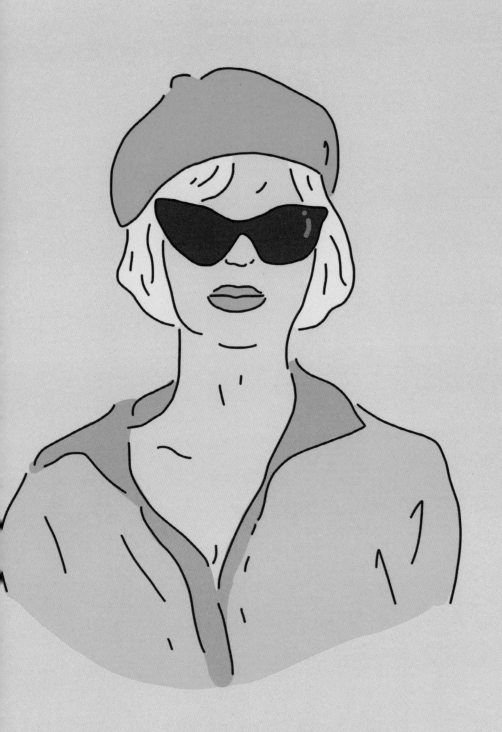

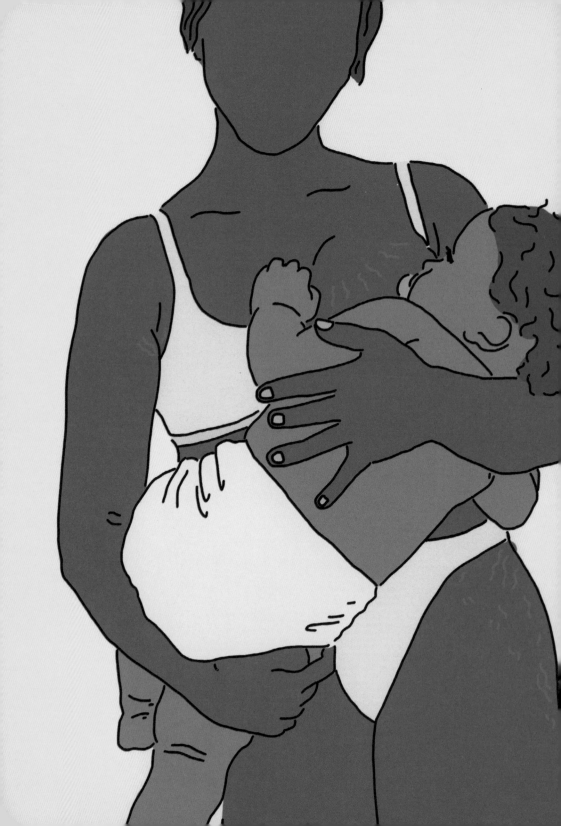

BREASTFEEDING IS A PERSONAL DECISION

Whether you decide to breastfeed or not, beware, the judgment is constant. If you choose not to breastfeed, you are immediately labeled a "shameful mother," who refuses her child the health benefits of breast milk. Breastfeeding carries many benefits for the baby and the mother, but it also takes an enormous physical and mental toll on the mother, which shouldn't be taken for granted. And then there are women who simply CAN'T breastfeed. And everything is made more difficult by society's unhealthy gaze that always sexualizes female breasts. "Cover that breast that I cannot see," said Molière, a still-present sentiment. Therefore, breastfeeding in public can be a challenge. And since we are talking about difficulties, the pressure of being the only one who can feed the child is not a walk in the park. Can you imagine being a breastfeeding mother while working? While it can be logistically challenging, some employers may refuse to help, so some women end up without jobs. It's complicated, I told you! So, let's stop with the taboos and judgment, once and for all!

#NORMALIZEBREASTFEEDING

#STOPSEXUALIZINGFEMALEBREASTS

#BREASTFEEDINGISAPERSONALCHOICE

You should be able to choose whether you breastfeed or not without pressure or judgment.

MENOPAUSE: HELLO, WHO'S THERE?

We don't talk about menopause often, perhaps because it's not a very "sexy" topic in a world that puts youth on a pedestal. It's the moment when you say goodbye to your cycle forever! Apparently, it's not an easy experience, and the way it's described makes it sound like punishment. "Now take your things and get out of here with your menopause! It's over, you're on your way to old age. Condemned to endless hot flashes, fatigue, night sweats, hair falling out, and a sad sex life. . . ." Wow! What illness is this? Ah, no—in fact, it's just a natural part of the life of a woman (and trans men and nonbinary and intersexual people). Just as it's true that a woman's meaning in life is not to procreate, a woman's life doesn't end with menopause. How crazy is that?

No more periods. If I think about the pain they give me, I think that's cause for celebration. Menopause should be celebrated!

#ANORMALPARTOFAGING
#ANEWLIFESTEP   #MATURING
#FREEDOM   #AGING

Pop the champagne! Menopause has arrived! No more periods!

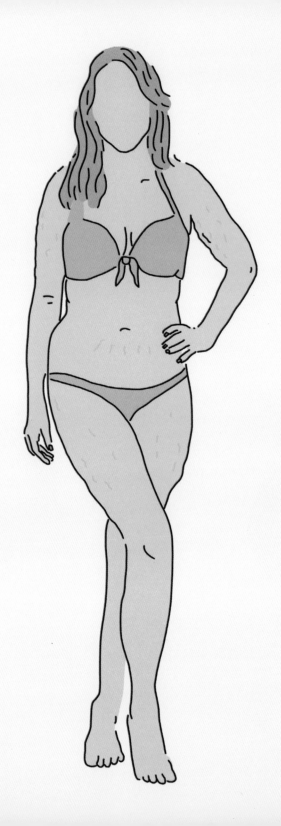

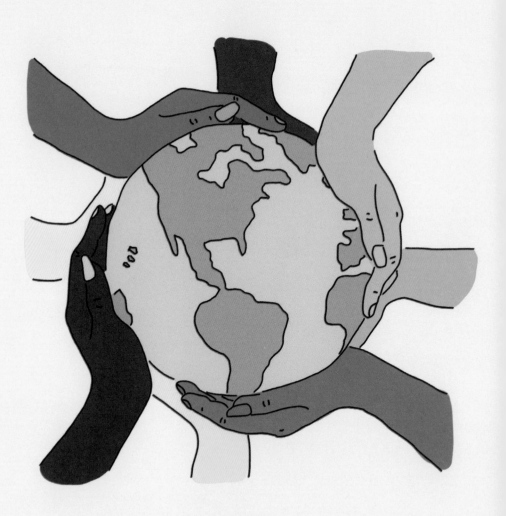

Chapter 7

. . . . .

Society: All Together Now

. . . . .

We are pigeonholed, male and female, as soon as we are born
(sometimes even before!). Our entire lives are steered in a certain
direction. We are bound to certain toys, certain colors, then certain
activities, certain studies, a certain level of freedom in imagining
ourselves . . . and behind these stereotypes is an enormous message:
equality doesn't exist. So here's the goal: no more standards!
And no more patriarchy. I realize achieving this is complicated,
but do we want a better world or not?

YOU DON'T HAVE TO BE
SMALL
OR LIMIT YOUR
RANGE
TO MAKE
OTHERS
FEEL
COMFORTABLE

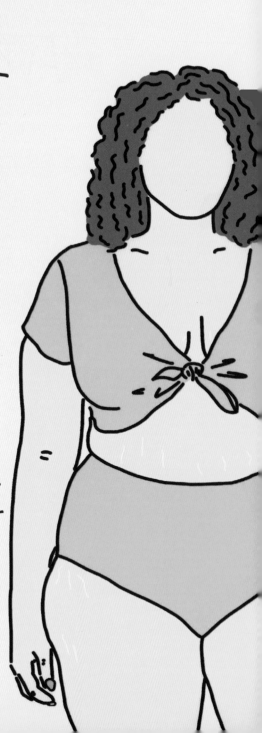

FREEDOM: TIMES ARE CHANGING

I don't want to be revolutionary, or even anxiety-inducing, but I think our freedoms are slowly being nibbled away. I don't want to reach a point in which we are scrutinized for our every move. Imagine if every time you bought a sex toy, your bank sent a notification to the seller.

"Ma'am, how is it possible that you bought three sex toys in the past week?"

"That's strange, it must be an error! You know women don't like sex!"

Fortunately, even though the battle for some freedoms is already under way, we are not backing down, like with women's rights and the right to abortion. We don't have to be activists, but we can't be indifferent toward the battles that affect us and our future. We must not be lazy when it comes to our freedoms. The freedom to think and live as we like and with whom we like—it's simple, but we still have to fight!

#MYLIFE

#UNCONDITIONALFREEDOM

Freedom has no price. But if we aren't careful, soon we won't know what it means anymore.

PRINCESSES: ONCE UPON A CLICHÉ . . .

Today, the passage of time allows me to see a moralist message that fed the machine in princess stories. A poor girl imprisoned by a "bad guy" waits to be freed by Prince Charming. Then there's the famous redemptive kiss. From a distance, the story is completely changed and the prejudice becomes clear. "But Mom, I thought a rich prince would have come looking for me and would have loved me forever! So why did unemployed Adrian eventually dump me?" Maybe I'm exaggerating, but the princess trope is truly depressing. It's about being beautiful so you can snatch a prince who will solve all your problems, as if we can't do anything for ourselves but try to please a man. I'm not saying we have to stop watching *Sleeping Beauty*, but we should pay more attention to the messages we are conveying to children and explain to them that they're not realistic. In any case, that's not the only option we have.

#NOTYOURPRINCESS

#ICANDOITBYMYSELF

#RELATIONSHIPBETWEENEQUALS

The princess trope is over, and we are better for it.

IF YOU'RE LOOKING
FOR A PERSON
WHO WILL
CHANGE
YOUR LIFE

LOOK IN
THE
MIRROR

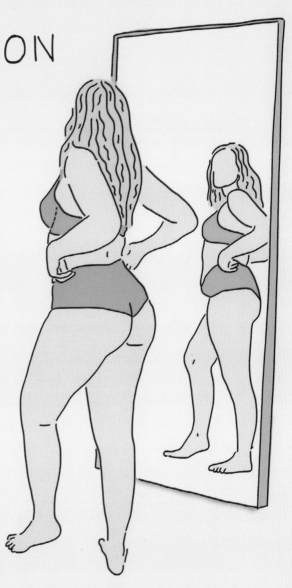

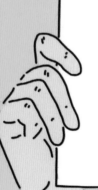

LET'S USE OUR STRENGTH TO MAKE CHANGE

THE ART OF TEACHING WHAT IS GOOD AND JUST

The line that divides education, expectations, and conditioning is very thin. Personally, I think we should reimagine education from top to bottom. Because our education system is made for the elite and protecting their privileges, and since we blur intelligence and knowledge, it won't be easy. We aren't even close. If we then add the fact that we spark competition between children from a young age, we can see the catastrophe emerging on the horizon. We are not taught to know ourselves, but rather to compare ourselves to others. But we aren't made for the same things. If we were taught to know ourselves, we would know what is good for us. And if we weren't pinned to certain roles, we would have more opportunities and would gain time. We are conditioned from childhood; and when we finally realize this, we spend time stripping away that conditioning. Isn't that a shame?

#REIMAGINETHEEDUCATIONSYSTEM

#STOPCONDITIONING

Fight for education that helps us—all of us—bloom.

A CAREER IS A RIGHT, NOT AN OBLIGATION

Why is it that the word *career* feels like a blow to the head? The word struck me when I first set foot in the music industry at seventeen years old. It still sounds just as mentally torturous as the day my producer, that large, imposing man, gave me an ultimatum, forcing me to choose between my "career" and my partner. Maybe that's because he made me believe that the contract was based on my youth or, in his words, my "purity." Or because he locked me in an office to prevent me from seeing my boyfriend. Or because it cost me financially *and* emotionally to get away from him after he made me sign the worst contracts with the promise of helping my career take off. All these reasons make me hate that word. The fight for equality goes on, but I am still worried for young and vulnerable girls who want to start their careers. When you have no experience, you don't always have the courage to say no, and that's dangerous.

#CAREERSWITHOUTPRESSURE

#STOPHARRASSMENT

A career is good, but not at any price!

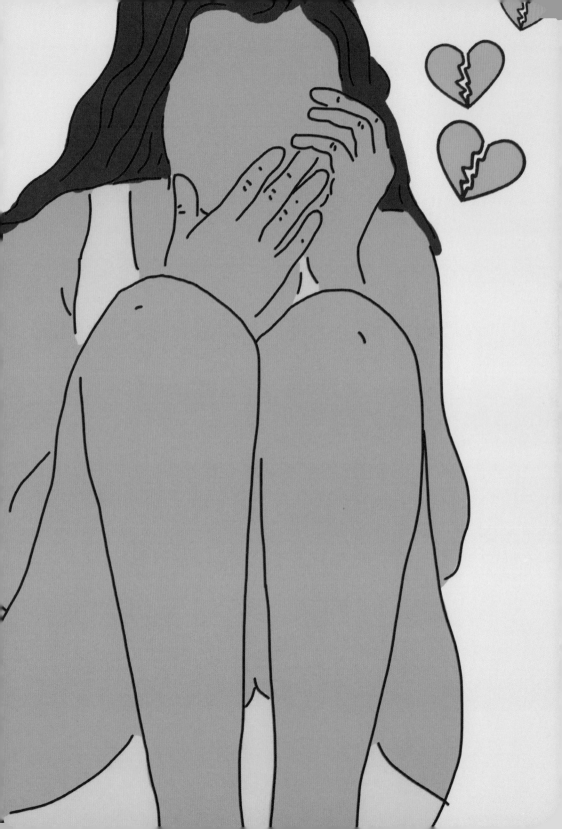

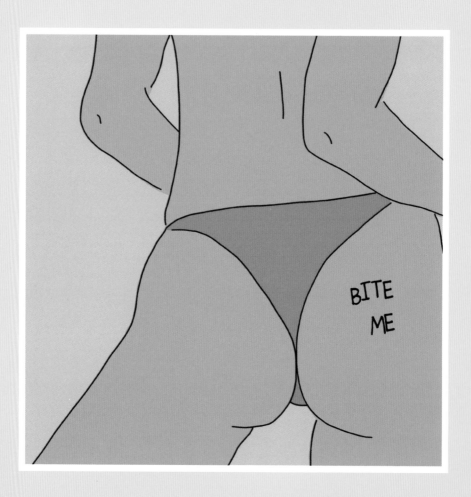

SEX SELLS ANYTHING

Oh, really? We live in a sexualized society? I hadn't noticed. I hadn't noticed that the photos on Instagram that perform the best are those of super-sexy young girls. Models in swimsuits with their legs apart. I hadn't noticed that on TikTok it's the same, but with one addition: they are dancing.

I know that it's not pictures of landscapes that work best on social media. Sexualization sells! It sells lotions, cars, marmalades, anything. It is a technique as old as time that still works today. The desire for a product is associated with sexual desire. Of course, it's always the female body that's sexualized. This custom has become a part of our society, and it's a tragic reality. But enough, don't you think? Aren't we tired of this hyper-consumerist society? Are we afraid we will get bored? There are so many things we could do, like grab a coffee or take a walk—and for once, leave your phone at home.

#STOPSEXUALIZATION
#NONCOMPULSIVEPLEASURE

If we consumed less, we'd have more time for other things.

BEWARE OF CENSORSHIP!

Censorship. Just the word makes me tense up. It embodies all the hypocrisy that exists in our society. On the one hand, we use sex to sell more; on the other, we completely censor the body. Instagram has become indispensable for my work as a healer, so I don't want to bite the hand that feeds me, but what a challenge . . . it's puritanical and conservative. I always have to pay attention to EVERYTHING I post, blurring, pixelating, and blocking every female nipple (though male ones are OK) for fear of being reported for yet another picture, which kills the whole project and five and a half years of work. I have already lost my Facebook page, a sneaky and unfair penalty from the men of Silicon Valley. It's terrifying! I was careful, but did I miss part of a nipple somewhere? How scandalous! The penalties hit left and right with no warning, and you find yourself helpless before this totalitarian censorship. So now I'm lying low.

It is the triumph of hypocrisy when we think of the reach of sexist, violent, fatphobic, and homophobic comments that incite hate and are never censored on Instagram. Nope, it's female bodies in the crosshairs of the Internet police. The body that doesn't adhere to the famous standards: fat rolls and body hair, these sorts of things. This censorship is not just crude, but it also has a real impact on marginalized, feminist, queer, trans, and sex work minorities.

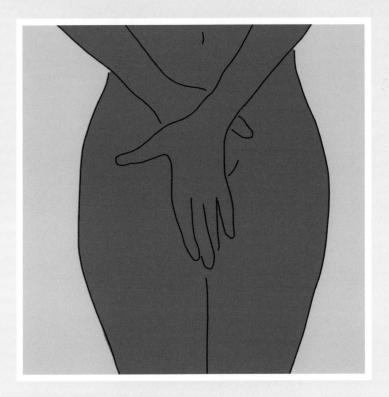

And if we think about it, social media has very precise methods for controlling and "cleansing" their platforms, with employees who are forced to look through whole swaths of content, including things of unspeakable violence. It's certainly effective, but it leaves a mark on these underpaid employees.

#STOPCENSORINGWOMENSBODIES

#FREEDOMOFEXPRESSION

#FREETHENIPPLE

Censorship of the female body shows how deeply rooted the objectification of women is in our society.

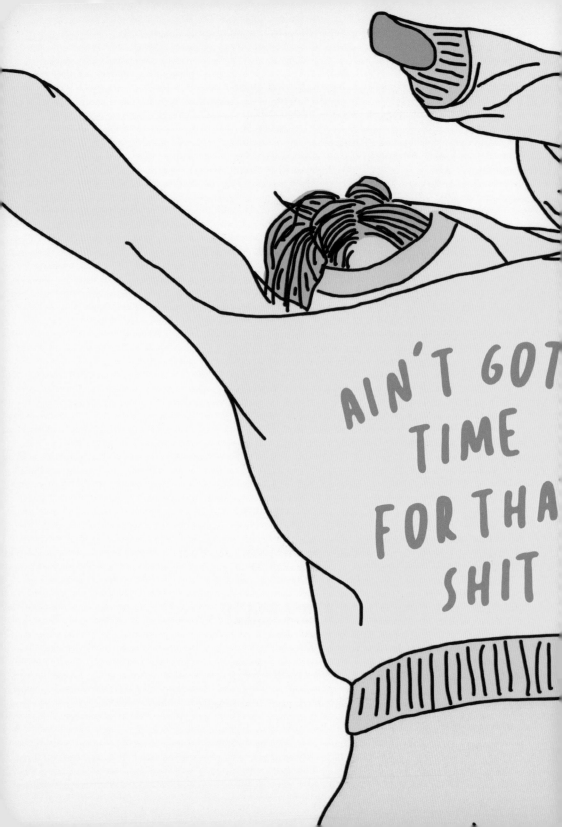

NO COMMENT

Welcome to the age of social media, which is a haven for trolls and mean comments. Why take your time to think when you can just write whatever comes to your head? And since they're sitting behind a screen, they're able to anonymously say awful things. When comments are kind, that's great. But we also see hate, jealously, cruelty, and just stupid comments. And this can cause serious damage to those on the receiving end. Words can destroy people. Before writing a comment, we should ask ourselves why we are doing it. If it is kind, there is little risk of negative repercussions...unless you're giving your two cents to your ex who has started a life with someone else. Too many people write from impulse, and it's sad when negative emotions gain the upper hand. It's best to just turn off the computer and go for a walk.

#NOCOMMENT #BEHINDTHESCREEN
#SPITTINGVENOM
#WORDSHAVEWEIGHT

In the game of comments, you could meet someone who manages their words better than you.
Being kind doesn't hurt.

THE FIGHT FOR EQUALITY

As long as there's something to fight for, the battle has not yet been won. And as for gender equality, we aren't there yet. Women continue to earn less, are judged more, and endure injustice. The situation for women on the job market is still more fragile than it is for men. Therefore, we must deal with sexism every day so that women are respected and not treated like objects. Slowly we are starting to see hope, but we need radical change to really see the light. Salary equality would be a nice win, but it wouldn't change the situation. If we really want to change things, we need to reimagine the structure of society to be built on equality. Why should we insist on carrying on with a failing system? That is the question. Byeee!

#THEFIGHTCONTINUES #EQUALITY
#AJUSTANDINCLUSIVEFUTURE #LETSGO

We have a long road ahead to create
a just and inclusive future so that a woman
can really "have it all" (and not be paid
less than a man).

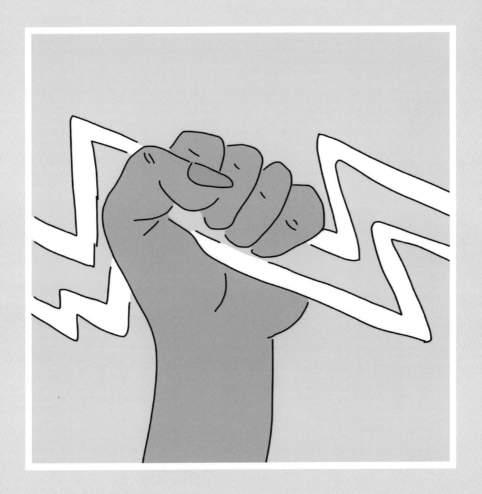

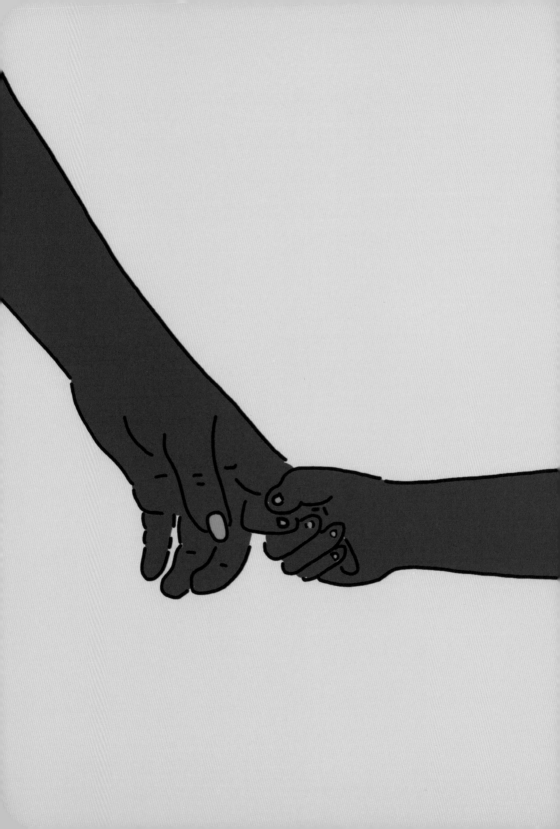

CAREGIVING

In many cases, women are expected to take care of everything and deal with every emergency! It's a heavy social burden that persists in many families. Luckily, the era of advertising in which a housewife with an apron and a big smile is center stage selling some detergent or appliance is over. Thank god. This was a big step forward for humanity. Are women really only interested in dealing with domestic matters and children? This is still an imposed standard.

Altruism is not based on gender. We all have the capacity for it. But poor cis men, they are victims of horrible hormonal fluctuations, especially PMS, which basically makes them unstable and aggressive, and therefore incapable of handling children . . . oh, oops . . . sorry, my bad!

#DONTFORGETYOURSELF

#TAKECAREOFOTHERS   #BEKIND

#TAKECAREOFYOURSELF

Altruism has no gender.

MONEY, MONEY, MONEY

My wallet is lucky I'm not a shopaholic. But instead of blaming sixteen-year-olds with a shopping addiction, we should reimagine the way things are sold (a.k.a. to push overconsumption). Commerce must be more just and equitable, but not just in commercials. I'm talking to brands that dominate the market: stop pretending. Be honest and respectful toward your employees and the society of developing countries where workers are exploited.

We, too, must stop pretending that this situation doesn't exist. As consumers, we can say something. If we stop buying, they will stop selling. And with our small amount of buying power, we can buy less and better. The idea is not to kill the economy, but to sound the alarm bells. We don't need strawberries all year round. We can experiment with a better system in which personal actualization doesn't coincide with materialistic success, based on how much you earn and own.

#CONSUMELESSANDBETTER

#ECORESPONSIBILITY

#STOPOVERCONSUMPTION

It is time to consume less and more intelligently, to think in the long term for a more balanced world that is less focused on profit.

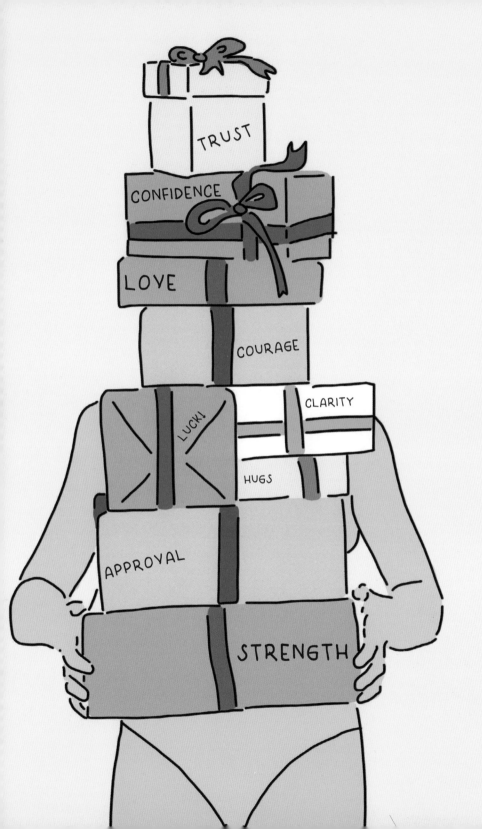

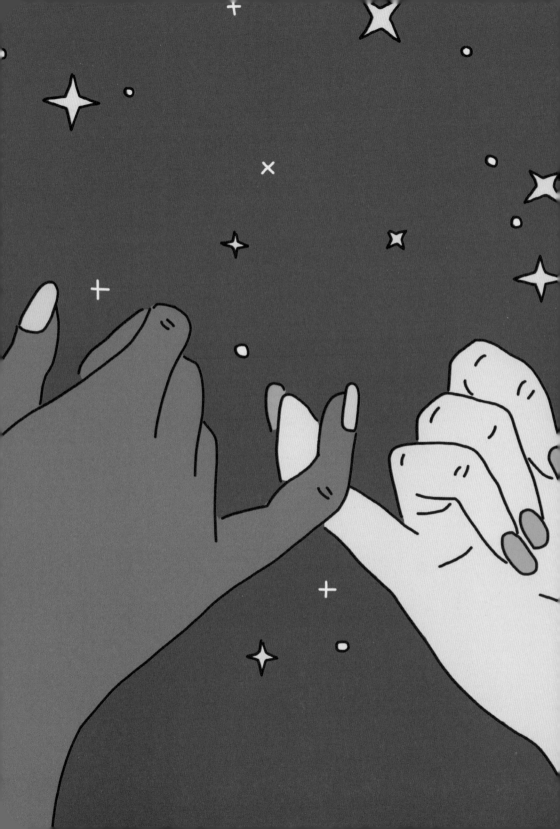

SISTERHOOD AGAINST OPPRESSION

Sisterhood is a bond of female solidarity that, in response to the patriarchy, allowed us to take great steps forward for our rights. The priority is to be united and unanimous in fighting injustices and sexist violence. One for all and all for one! It might seem cheesy, but uniting our voices is an outstanding strength in a culture that pushes us to judge, criticize, and underestimate each other. The internalized misogyny that still echoes in our heads is the product of a "divide and conquer" society.

But if we let ourselves get carried away with competition, the road to gender equality will be long. The more we are united, the stronger our voices will be. The right to vote, abortion, and equal pay: we have won a few battles, but there's still much to do, especially for queer, BIPOC, and disabled women. We need to stand together for the rights of all! It's time to stop oppressing each other and start solving everything together. Let's go!

#SISTERHOOD   **#TOGETHERWEARESTRONGER**
#COMPREHENSIONNOTCOMPETITION
#STOPINTERNALIZEDMISOGYNY

Don't let internalized misogyny
pit us against each other.
Support your sisters.

ART: A MAGICAL TOOL FOR COMBATING STIGMA

Art is often a representation of our thoughts or deep feelings, and it incites emotions and important reflections in society. It is also an incredible form of therapy, because it allows you to express your vision or story without fear. We can transmit a shocking or subtle message, but the viewer will perceive and interpret it in their own way. This is the magic of art.

We know that many women were excluded from "artistic" professions (since weaving, embroidery, woodworking, and pottery aren't real art, right?) until the twentieth century. But without a *female narrative*, we find ourselves prisoners of the male gaze, which objectifies the female body, perpetuating false ideas about us. There should be no gender divides in art. But there are different perspectives, and the existence of oppression and inequality makes it necessary for women to have their own space to counterbalance the dialogue.

Unfortunately, I believe art alone is not enough to change the world. One reason is that art has become a business; unfortunately, money often ruins things. Art shouldn't seek commercial success. It should be a pure and personal journey of initiation, a search for the self and a connection to others.

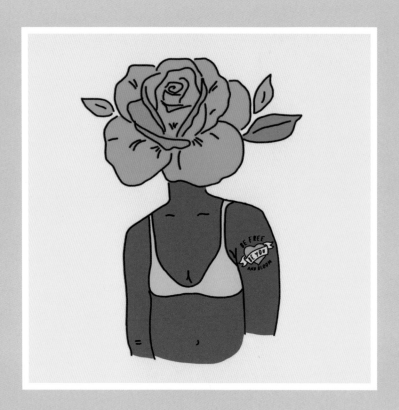

#FEMALEGAZE   #GIVESPACE
#REPRESENTATIONCOUNTS
#REFLECTIONFORSOCIETY
#ARTTHERAPY

Art is a personal journey through emotions and
deep thoughts. It must include female and
non-binary perspectives.

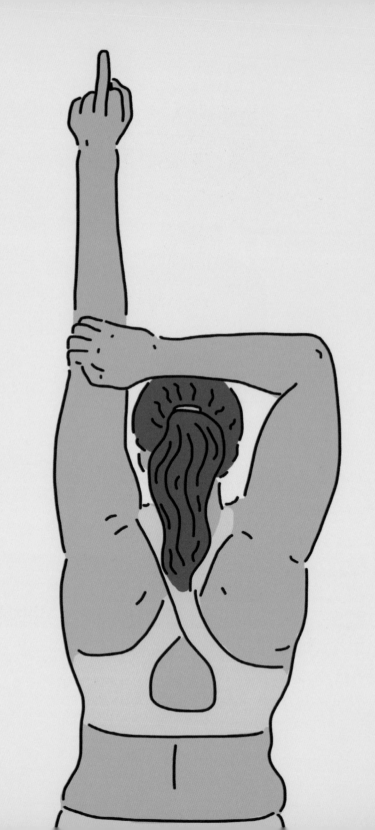

FAREWELL, PATRIARCHY

The patriarchy is a system based on the fact that power is held by . . . drumroll, please . . . oooh! suspense . . . the wait is killing me . . . yes, MEN!! And with the explicit exclusion of women. Here's an excellent definition I found on the Internet: "The masculine occupies both that which is superior and universal, dividing everyone else into groups based on sex, gender, sexual orientation, ethnicity, and social class." I've said it since the beginning: the patriarchy is a nightmare, and it has been going on for far too long. A society based on such unequal privilege can only lead to oppression and discrimination and cannot function correctly. But eliminating it is not easy. Today the patriarchy continues to cling tight to its hold like a clam to its shell! It's everywhere, insidious. In education, in our lives, in media. Only by becoming aware and acting can we manage to change things, little by little, for a more just society. Onward!

#SMASHTHEPATRIARCHY

#NEWSOCIETY   **#EQUALITY**

#TOOMANYMACHOMEN

Put on your boots and stomp out
the patriarchy, step by step.
You will be headed for
a better world.

Cheers Baby!

· · · · · ·

The Menstrual Cycle: It's the World Turning

· · · · · ·

The menstrual cycle is incredible. It usually starts when a person with a uterus is between eleven and thirteen years old. It begins an average of every twenty-eight days, with the period lasting between three and seven days, all for the next thirty or forty years. Don't worry, I'm not going to give you a science lesson, I just want to insist that we can be proud of ourselves for managing it. Sometimes it's tiring. "Great . . . my period arrived," we grumble sarcastically. And each month it starts again. . . .

hey there, handsome!

PERIODS! "I SAID HEY! WHAT'S GOING ON?"

My period took forever to arrive. When my best friend in elementary school one day at recess announced that she was a "woman" at eleven years old, I hoped that I would become one soon too. How naïve! I watched my sisters and imagined what might happen to me. They got theirs at thirteen and fourteen years old, so I figured I would also get mine later than my BFF! But I never would have thought it would take so long! You might not believe me, but my period showed up when I no longer believed it would come: on my eighteenth birthday! About time!! Before then, I avoided the subject in the locker room for fear of being considered an alien! Being different: no, thanks! I waited patiently for the day to arrive, and I then entered the world of the divine force of menstrual blood, but also that of taboo, shame, and premenstrual syndrome (PMS)! A little bonus I'd been missing in my life.

#PEEPO   #ABOUTTIME
#ENTERWOMANHOOD

The arrival of your period is a special and unique moment.

PERIODS ARE RED, NOT BLUE

It's the cycle of life, and yet it remains a shameful topic. We should be able to talk about it freely, because it's a natural, almost banal, phenomenon. But we live in a patriarchal society (once again), and blood that drips from the uterus is disturbing, much more so than the blood in gory films. Periods are an ancestral taboo, something that was labeled as "disgusting" and that should be hidden. Therefore, in advertising and commercials for sanitary products, a BLUE liquid has been used to represent period blood. What a bizarre idea! We all know that menstrual blood is red, even *bright* red. It makes you think. Advertising also boasts of the refreshing qualities of their products, as if having your period was dirty.

This topic has been removed from the discussion, and so rarely represented in culture, that society has never stopped feeling offended by the slightest glimpse of menstrual blood. Let's stop being ashamed of our bodies and how they function!

#STOPTABOOS

#NORMALIZEMENSTRATION

#SHOCKOFMENSTRUALBLOOD

Is menstrual blood really scarier than violence and war?

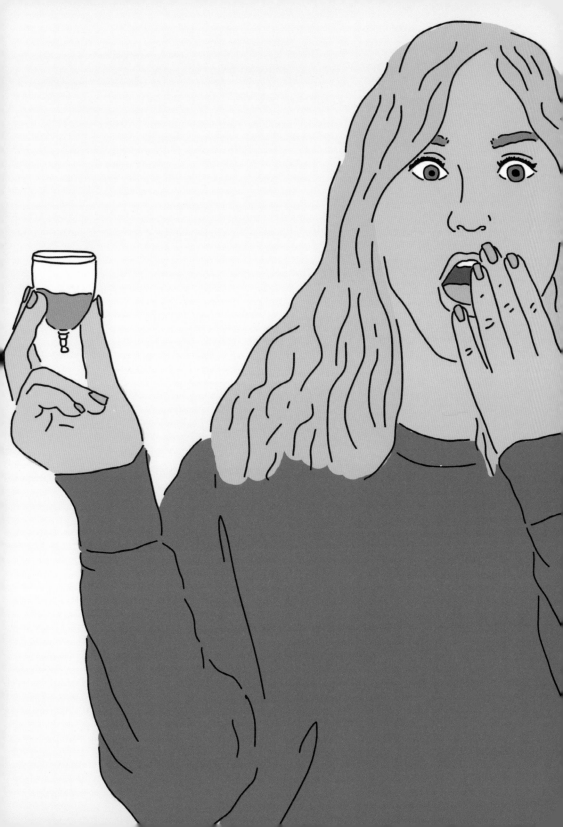

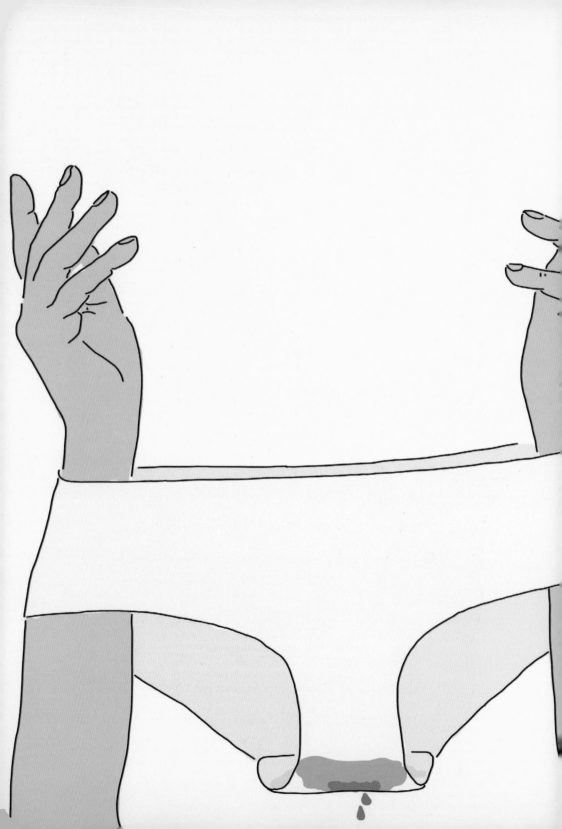

NOT ONLY WOMEN GET PERIODS

This is understandably a sensitive subject. Having a period is not enjoyable, and much suffering comes from them—taboos, cramps, PMS—and we must deal with social, physical, and financial consequences. It's a burden. Therefore, it makes sense that we defend it as a phenomenon that regards women.

BUT . . . there's a but . . . being inclusive doesn't hurt. And having a cycle doesn't necessarily make you a "woman." It is a natural phenomenon for many cis women, but let's not forget that trans men and nonbinary and intersexual individuals also have them. And there are a number of reasons that some cis women do not experience a natural menstrual cycle, but that doesn't make them less than in any way. Let's try living in harmony with everyone around us. Let's stop believing in a binary world, men on one side and women on the other. Even if we can't understand the motivations and journey of each person, we must respect them. It's that simple.

#LGBTQ   #QUEER   #NONBINARY
#TRANSMEN   #INCLUSIVE
#MENSTRUATIONANDGENDER   #INCLUSION

Let's include everyone with a uterus in discussions about menstruation.

BLEEDING: A CRIME SCENE ON YOUR CLOTHES

Hello, spotting! Who hasn't found blood on their sheets or underwear? But we don't talk about it. It's shameful. Once, I got so much blood on a dress, an obviously shameful and disgusting experience, that I preferred throwing it out to trying to clean it. That's a bit crazy, don't you think? But it's been implied that when we get our period, we must "protect" ourselves. That's a strong statement. *Protect* ourselves? From what? Well, from total shame. Because if we have our period, the most important thing is that others not know it. That would be . . . wait for it . . . SHAMEFUL!

But who decided that periods are dirty? And why should we be ashamed? Our vagina and vulva are incredible machines that are self-cleaning, and we should be proud of them! There's no reason to be ashamed of such a normal experience.

#LETITFLOW   #ITSNATURAL
#DISMANTLESHAME
#OOPSNOTAGAIN

Fifty percent of the global population has them. It's normal! Be proud of your menstrual cycle.

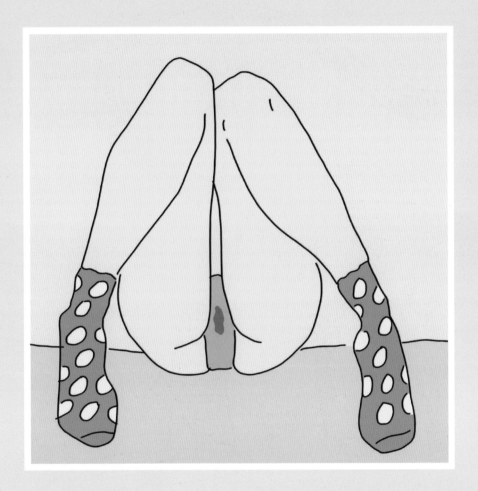

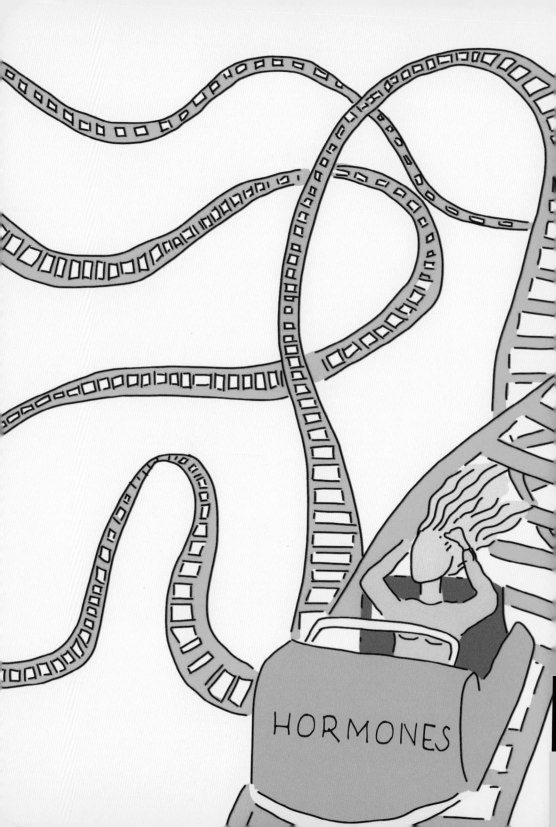

PMS: A HORMONAL ROLLER COASTER

Many women—nine out of ten—feel a wave of anxiety and dark thoughts a few days before their cycle. It's an unpleasant sensation that can upset us, and it's called premenstrual syndrome, or PMS. But no one teaches us how to manage it! Every time, I get irritable, almost aggressive. And I naturally am very shy and gentle . . . so strange! The smallest observation can set me off and push me to question many aspects of my life! My poor partner always ends up in the middle of it. Then, after a couple of days, he realizes: "Oh, so you didn't want to leave me, you just had PMS! So I can unpack my bags then?"

PMS is a strange phenomenon. For a few days, I have crazy and terrifying dreams that seem straight out of a Tarantino film. It's a time of hypersensitivity that puts us in touch with our fears and anxieties. But, after that, we become very creative, because pain and anxiety breed inspiration.

#HORMONESATWAR

#ROLLERCOASTER   #EMOTIONS

Our emotions take a ride on the PMS roller coaster, and they manifest in different ways.

ACCESS TO MENSTRUAL PRODUCTS FOR ALL

Some women use a menstrual cup, but it doesn't work for everyone. I started by using pads and tampons, then I realized how harmful they are for the planet and my body. It really worried me. So I opted for other solutions. I love period underwear. They are the most comfortable and best for the environment. In any case, whatever we choose is expensive. In addition to being a topic too shameful to openly discuss, periods are also a source of inequality on a social and economic level. Because it costs to have a period! Yup, you have to budget for it. We shouldn't have to decide between eating and bleeding. That's where the fight for eliminating the tampon tax started: all sanitary products are considered nonessential items and therefore carry a higher tax. "Period poverty" is still a taboo, like everything related to periods, so we must fight to make menstrual products accessible for everyone with a menstrual cycle.

#FREEPERIODPRODUCTS

#ENDPERIODPOVERTY

#ACCESSTOPERIODPRODUCTS

#EQUALACCESS

Period justice is a right, not a luxury.

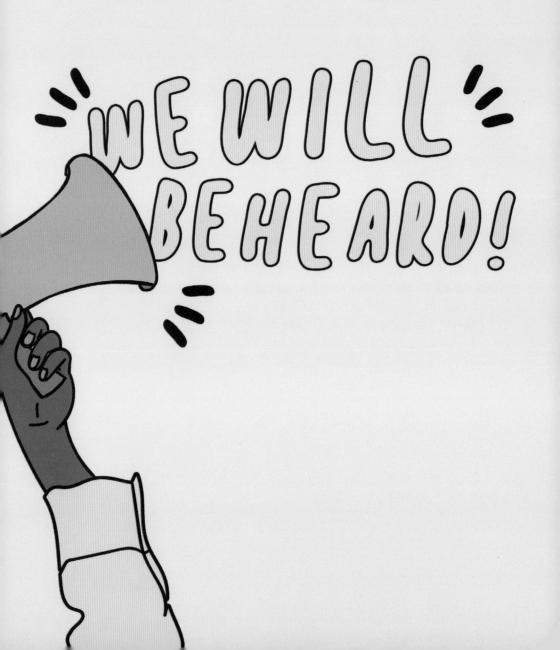

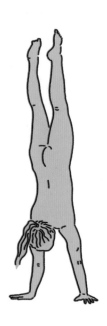

Laetitia Duveau

Laetitia Duveau is part of a new generation of multitasking women who adapt to a changing world, and she has diversified her knowledge as much as possible. An author, composer, and musician, she became an art curator in 2016 in Berlin, where she established a home for four fruitful and intense years. There, she started *Curated by GIRLS*, a platform that promotes the diversity of women through art, offering visibility to artists without censorship or compensation. Today it is known worldwide. She recently moved to the mystical town of Sintra, Portugal, where she works insatiably on a variety of projects under the nickname Little Voice, such as singing in the indie-pop duo Free Dom Dom and dancing professionally.

Bridget Moore

Bridget Moore is an artist from Los Angeles more commonly known by the pseudonym Handsome Girl. Her work mainly consists of digital illustrations and is focused on themes of intersectional feminism, body positivity and female empowerment. She is very passionate about the movement for inclusion and representation, and her goal is to ensure all women of any background or experience are seen and heard. Moore began drawing as therapy for an eating disorder she had been battling for years. This is how she came to celebrate the beauty of her own body and those of other women, and to depict different shapes, forms and experiences that manifest beauty.

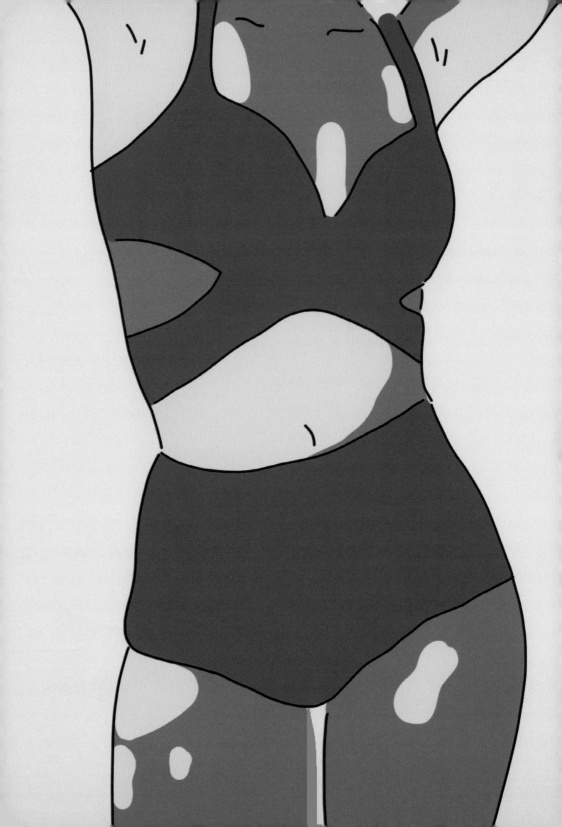